Creative Counselling

by the same author

Doodle Your Worries Away
A CBT Doodling Workbook for Children Who Feel Worried or Anxious
Tanja Sharpe
ISBN 978 1 78775 790 5
eISBN 978 1 78775 791 2

CBT Doodling for Kids
50 Illustrated Handouts to Help Build Confidence and
Emotional Resilience in Children Aged 6–11
Tanja Sharpe
ISBN 978 1 78592 537 5
eISBN 978 1 78775 017 3

of related interest

The CBT Art Activity Book
100 illustrated handouts for creative therapeutic work
Jennifer Guest
ISBN 978 1 84905 665 6
eISBN 978 1 78450 168 6

Counselling Skills for Working with Trauma
Healing From Child Sexual Abuse, Sexual Violence and Domestic Abuse
Christine Sanderson
ISBN 978 1 84905 326 6
eISBN 978 0 85700 743 8

Effective Self-Care and Resilience in Clinical Practice
Dealing with Stress, Compassion Fatigue and Burnout
Edited by Sarah Parry
Foreword by Paul Gilbert
ISBN 978 1 78592 070 7
eISBN 978 1 78450 331 4

CREATIVE COUNSELLING

Creative Tools and Interventions to Nurture Therapeutic Relationships

Tanja Sharpe

Foreword by Suzanne Alderson

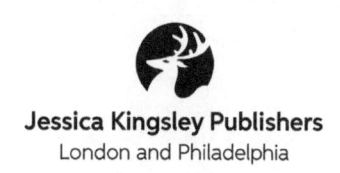

Jessica Kingsley Publishers
London and Philadelphia

First published in Great Britain in 2022 by Jessica Kingsley Publishers
An imprint of Hodder & Stoughton Ltd
An Hachette Company

5

Copyright © Tanja Sharpe 2022

The right of Tanja Sharpe to be identified as the Author of the Work has been asserted by her in accordance with the Copyright, Designs and Patents Act 1988.

Foreword © Suzanne Alderson 2022

Front cover image source: Creative Counsellors. The cover image is for illustrative purposes only, and any person featuring is a model.

All rights reserved. No part of this publication may be reproduced, stored in a retrieval system, or transmitted, in any form or by any means without the prior written permission of the publisher, nor be otherwise circulated in any form of binding or cover other than that in which it is published and without a similar condition being imposed on the subsequent purchaser.

There are supplementary materials which can be downloaded from https://library.jkp.com/redeem for personal use with this programme, but may not be reproduced for any other purposes without the permission of the publisher.

A CIP catalogue record for this title is available from the
British Library and the Library of Congress

ISBN 978 1 83997 018 4
eISBN 978 1 83997 017 7

Printed and bound by CPI Group (UK) Ltd, Croydon, CR0 4YY

Jessica Kingsley Publishers' policy is to use papers that are natural, renewable and recyclable products and made from wood grown in sustainable forests. The logging and manufacturing processes are expected to conform to the environmental regulations of the country of origin.

Jessica Kingsley Publishers
Carmelite House
50 Victoria Embankment
London EC4Y 0DZ

www.jkp.com

Contents

Acknowledgements 9

Foreword by Suzanne Alderson 11

Embracing Your Creative Spark – My Heart-Powered Wish for You . 15

1. Introduction to Creative Counselling 17
    What is Creative Counselling?   17
    The Create Circle Approach   21
    Can Creative Interventions be Integrated into Any Core
        Counselling Model?   24
    What if I am Not Creative?   24
    Why Creative Counselling Now?   25

2. Create the Right Environment 29
    Exploring Different Creative Counselling Environments   29
    Indoor Therapy Rooms   31
    Neurodiversity and Room Lighting   31
    Sourcing Resources for Your Therapy Room   32
    Creating Diverse Therapy Spaces   35
    Storing Resources in Your Therapy Room   37
    Carrying Resources as a Mobile Counsellor   40
    Virtual Counselling – Working Creatively Online   41
    Working Creatively in the Outdoors and Walk-and-Talk Counselling   47
    Creatively Working with Nature as a Co-Therapist   50
    Reflections   53

3. Relationship and Grounding 55
   The First Creative Connection – Your Marketing   55
   Creative Additions to Contracting   57
   Taking Your Client's Lead – 'Pace and Check'   58
   Working Creatively with Grounding Tools   60
   Mind, Body, Feelings and Intuition (MBFI)   68
   Check In, Creative Process, Check Out   70
   Knowing When to Pivot or Shift Exercise   71
   Reflections   77

4. Engage and Evaluate 79
   Creative Interventions to Help Engage the Client in the Goals-Setting Process   79
   Creative Assessments   79
   My Life Circle   80
   Working with Number-Range Assessments   81
   Sand-Tray Families and Relationships   82
   A Hopes-and-Dreams Board   82
   Evaluating Triggers   84
   Doodling, Sketching and Drawing   84
   Nature Metaphors   85
   From-Here-to-There Exercise   85
   Tools Timeline   86
   Reflections   90

5. Creative Activities and Interventions 91
   Working Creatively with Sound in the Counselling Room   92
   Poetry as a Creative Intervention   98
   Incorporating Role Play in the Counselling Room   100
   Creative Art Interventions in Counselling   103
   Creative Therapeutic Journaling   110
   Working Creatively with Mandalas   114
   Working Creatively with Clay in the Counselling Room   118
   Working Creatively with Puppets   123
   Working Creatively with Stones in the Counselling Room   127
   Working with Creative Visualization in the Counselling Room   132

Working Creatively with Nesting Dolls in the Counselling Room	137
Working Therapeutically with Characters, Fairy Tales and Stories	139
Working Therapeutically with Sand	141
Working Creatively with Empty Chair Cards	143
Reflections	146

6. Take Time to Reflect 147

Exploring Reflective Practice	147
Our Roots Influence our Reflections	149
Reflecting through Mind, Body, Feelings and Intuition (MBFI Reminder)	152
Tuning In	153
Exploring Angles and Perspectives	154
Validating and Holding Feelings, Emotions and Experiences	155
Five Creative Reflection Approaches	157
Reflections	159

7. Endings and New Beginnings 161

Exploring Endings in Creative Counselling	161
Planned Endings	162
Unplanned Endings	163
Contracting and Goal Setting	163
Confidentiality	164
Physical Space and Environment	165
Storing Client Work	166
Placing Symbols	167
Photographing Work	168
On Saying Goodbye to Our Clients at the End of Therapy	169
Reflections	174

8. Exploring the I in *CreatIvIty* 175

Finding Creative Inspiration	176
Four Ways to Find Creative Inspiration for *You*	177
Deepening Your Self-Awareness	178
Nurturing Your Own Creativity	182
20 Prompts to Boost Creativity for *You*	183

Counsellor Self-Care	188
Creative Counselling Community	197
Training and Confidence to Practise	198
Creative Supervision	199
Ethical Framework, Membership and Insurance	200
Bringing Creative Counselling to Your Organization	201

Extra Resources and Support	207
Downloads	207
Contact	207
Community	207

References	209

Index	213

Acknowledgements

I dedicate this book to all the incredible Creative Counsellors® who are inspiring change in the world, especially to our Creative Counsellors Community members, who have become family!

To my incredible Creative Counsellors team, a heartfelt thank you for this inspiring adventure we are on together. We have been a team for most of this community journey and there aren't enough thank yous in the world to recognize the contribution that you make to the Creative Counsellors Movement.

A huge thank you to *Suzanne*, who has been at my side night and day to support me throughout all my adventures in business, writing, dreaming and creating.

Thank you to my supervisor, *Joan*, who has been with me from the beginning of my counselling journey and always has an open door and a fresh perspective on the many challenges – personal and professional – that I bring to our sessions.

A special thanks to the following counsellors who have contributed by writing and sharing their unique interventions in this book:

Shelby Priestley
Kemi Omijeh
Masha Bennett
Rebecca Watson
Evie Sharpe
Caroline Peacock
Honorata Chorąży-Przybysz
Denise Richards

Cara Cramp
Rhiannon Davies
Tracy Dunning
Tara O'Kane
Lin Sharpe
Yasmin Shaheen-Zaffar
Gaynor Rimmer
Lisa Cromar

Foreword

SUZANNE ALDERSON

From a young age, being creative seemed to me to be the ultimate act of bravery and, sadly, one I wasn't brave enough for. That belief began when I was a child and it was something I held on to for far too many years. Looking back, it may well have been a perfectionist family member ridiculing and angrily fixing my far-from-perfect egg-box explorations. I'm sure my teacher's takedown of my 12-year-old self's proud painting of Mr Happy didn't help either. Nor did the tutor's laughter at my attempts at a hand-built cup at a weekend ceramics club.

I felt that I was being consistently and vociferously told that I wasn't creative and to just, please, give it up. No one seemed interested in the song in my heart or the verse in my mind. For my own protection, I listened to their truths and, over time, stopped floating away on visions of the books I would write, the spaces I would create and the beauty I could see. I was destined to live a prosaic life of pragmatism, devoid of creation. I would be a non-creator; someone who didn't make anything except, it seemed, a mess.

Some 40 years after that first judgement cemented a life view that if I wasn't technically competent at the visual arts, I couldn't be creative, I met someone who freed me from the need for permission to embrace the way creativity came to me and who showed me its power to unlock the beliefs and blockages that define the way we live our lives. As soon as Tanja and I connected as two of just 115 people selected by Facebook as their most meaningful community leaders in the world and placed on a programme of mentorship, training and support, I felt safe. I'd come home, and I knew we were starting a lifelong journey of connection, friendship and growth.

It wasn't just her open, natural, nurturing way, or the genuine interest she showed in my life and work, or the uncanny sense that I'd come home to a wonderful safe space that felt right whatever was going on in the world. It was a strange power that emanated from Tanja: a calmness, a compassion and a belief that everything we need is within us and is within our power, if we only allow ourselves to see it, feel it and, most importantly, create it.

Tanja taught me that *this* is real creativity. It doesn't have to be worthy of a place on the wall or even something you might want to keep in order to be creative or meaningful. The act of creating is where the magic happens, not the final output. The human compulsion is to make – to express ourselves through movement, whether that's our mouths speaking, our bodies moving or our minds flowing our needs through our hands and hearts. And her life's work is to enable us as people and practitioners to be brave enough to begin that journey of self-discovery and see how it can serve us and those we support to understand ourselves better.

Tanja talked me down from the narrative that had run through my life and my heart – that I was not creative – and she gently opened me up to the possibility that not only was I truly creative, but also that the belief in my creativity was mine alone to determine.

Tanja gently showed me that being creative wasn't something I did only when I had the acrylic paints out or when I set aside time. It is in the way I live my life; in how I deal with the sunshine and the fires; in the choices and changes I am in control of; in the way I think and problem solve.

Tanja has taught me that every one of us is creative if we only allow ourselves to explore it.

That we are creating in every moment and with every choice.

That craft does not equal creativity.

That creative competence doesn't equate to creative consciousness.

That we can all unlock that space that I thought was reserved for 'the artists' and by doing so unlock the emotions that we rationalize and compartmentalize far too quickly.

Tanja has encouraged and supported me to live a creative life and to live life creatively. And as the visionary and founder of a global movement of Creative Counsellors, I know she will encourage you too. Her own history and trauma, her experience, insight and learning, her open heart and creative mind, but most of all her unfailing belief, backed by years of experience and expertise, that we can all unlock the pain we hold within by allowing ourselves to explore our creative side are changing lives all over the world in the most nurturing and gentle way. A way that we need if we're going to make sense of the changes in our society and maintain our emotional wellbeing and long-term resilience.

Tanja pulls back the curtain on what creativity really is – its power to open us up, and empower us to believe in ourselves and our ability to grow and change. She reminds us that being creative is an act of curiosity, and a journey, not a destination. Creativity unlocks the layers of consciousness, and if we can approach counselling or our own connection to self through a lens of creativity, without judgement and with no expectation of outcome, it has alchemic powers of transformation.

I have been fortunate that Tanja is so generous with her gifts and time, and my community and charity has benefitted hugely from her efforts. She recently ran an eight-week intervention for the parents of young people with mental health issues whom we support called Creative Connections. The feedback from so many of the parents was that once they'd 'allowed' themselves to enjoy the process without focusing on the outcome, they gained a sense of joy they'd forgotten about and felt emotions they'd suppressed. Creativity takes us into a state of flow, and good – and challenging – things come from that.

As a counsellor, and as a human, I hope you take the approaches and techniques in this book and use them and share them and learn from them and grow from them. As someone who has had therapy, I'd ask you to approach your clients as if they were a 12-year-old who has had their painting laughed at, because being creative might not come easily at first. Encourage them – and yourself – to embrace the 'mistakes', because these are the lessons, and within them is what we seek and what is seeking us. Be gentle with them, and you, as you wrestle creativity from the conscious, certainty-seeking mind – and embrace the messy, beautiful experience of following a thought and making it real. Remind them that seeking to understand ourselves through creativity is an even braver act than creating for creating's sake; you really see your truest self through the mirror of creativity.

Tanja taught me that being creative is a brave pursuit but one that any of us is capable and worthy of. It is a powerful way to understand ourselves better and reconnect with the essence of our souls and selves. I sometimes wonder how my life might have been different had I met Tanja earlier, but knowing her now is more than enough. I am so grateful for the richness and acceptance she brings to me. She has elevated my understanding of myself and the potential I have to create change, harmony and love in my life, and I am deeply heartened and excited that she – and now you – have the tools and skills to support so many people to inner peace and calm through creativity.

Be brave with your creativity, so those you support can be brave too.

Suzanne Alderson
Founder and director of Parenting Mental Health charity and author of *Never Let Go: How to Parent Your Child Through Mental Illness*

Embracing Your Creative Spark – My Heart-Powered Wish for You

When we were born, we came into this world with new eyes and a radiating heart powered by a creative spark. Everything was an adventurous, playful and exciting quest. We learned to navigate life's moments through all our senses while we engaged with the world curiously and openly, trusting in the process wholeheartedly. We painted what we saw and what we felt, we dreamed without limitation and believed that everything was possible! We turned rocks into battleships and forests into fairy glens. We fought gremlins under bridges and built kingdoms made of blankets. Our entire life was constructed from metaphor and imagination, sparkling with colour and inspiration. But as we began to grow into our bodies and this human life, we started to understand what it was to know shame, guilt and failure, and with this came the inevitable time for us to learn to be in this world without imagination, without playfulness and curiosity. For many of us, our imaginations were belittled into believing that there was no place for daydreaming or adventure and that life was serious business with serious consequences. Our analytical brains were sparked into dominance and our creative spark became less and less until it was a tiny little ember waiting in the shadows of your heart to be reignited.

As you navigate the pages in this book, my wish for you is that you are able to find your way back to that creative spark that lives within your heart. To find inspiration in the playfulness, courage in the words and love in the meaning. That you are empowered to see yourself as the architect of your world and the magician in your counselling room, creating transformational and wild spaces for both you and your clients to roam free.

With love,
Tanja

Chapter 1

Introduction to Creative Counselling

WHAT IS CREATIVE COUNSELLING?

Creative Counselling combines talking therapies with creative interventions. As a model, Creative Counselling fundamentally respects a counsellor's core training model (such as Integrative, Person-Centred, Psychodynamic, Cognitive Behavioural Therapy or Transactional Analysis) and complements the core approach with creative interventions.

As an example, I am a Creative Integrative Counsellor and my core model is Integrative, combining Person-Centred, Psychodynamic and Cognitive Behavioural Therapy approaches with creative interventions.

Creative Counselling can include but is not limited to interventions like poetry, photography, art, nature, Mindfulness, role play, symbols, metaphor, sand, sound and play.

In my experience, many clients who come to therapy share that they find themselves looping in and out of the counselling process over the years because of not being able to find a way to fully communicate their experiences and feelings. There are many reasons for this, including:

- the effects of trauma and not being able to process them fully
- intense feelings and emotions around shame, fear and guilt
- fear of not saying the right thing or saying too much
- low self-esteem and the desire to please the therapist (people pleasing)
- not knowing where to begin or what to say

- knowing that they feel 'bad' but not knowing what they need
- feeling as though the words to describe how they are feeling or experiencing their life haven't been invented yet.

Research carried out by Lisa Cromar on behalf of Creative Counsellors shows that talking therapy is not always enough for clients (Cromar 2021), and in my experience, this means that counselling becomes exclusive to only those who can verbalize their words and emotions. Creative Counselling, on the other hand, empowers clients to express their words and emotions through any medium that feels right to them.

This is especially powerful for those clients who struggle with patterns of 'overanalysing' or 'overthinking' about what they might say, as it often helps clients to bring to the surface trapped feelings, emotions and new insight very quickly while working very deeply. It bypasses the process of overthinking and overanalysing. It works directly with the unconscious mind and will often take clients straight to the most important part of the work without a second thought. This helps us to work with key emotions, thoughts and behaviours without needing to get stuck in the story.

When we work from a Creative Counselling approach, we prioritize our clients' preferences, placing them at the core of the work and meeting them where they are at through their own lens (photography), witnessing their story playing out (role play) and experiencing their world through their own words (poetry). We give expression, movement, a voice, a shape, a symbol, a metaphor and colour to a client's experience, bringing it to life in a way that often words alone cannot.

Sometimes, words alone aren't enough in the therapy room, and in a little while we will explore a framework that really shines when we need a route to be able to facilitate therapy with clients that doesn't have to rely on words, one of the cornerstones of our *working-creatively approach*.

As Creative Counsellors, we think outside the box, scanning clients' interests and passions to tailor interventions to their individual needs, interests and goals. This can help to bridge the gap between the conscious and unconscious mind for clients, in turn creating new insight, growth and connection. Sometimes, it feels like the words to describe an emotion or experience haven't been invented yet and I have had my own experience of this during a sand-tray session with a therapist.

I am a survivor of childhood sexual abuse, and I didn't share my story and the associated shame that accompanied it until I was 18 years old. Like many survivors, I carried my secrets with me until it felt safe enough to unlock the door just a little and let someone in. At 18, I finally shared my story with my parents, and I never spoke of this again until my counselling training. During my training, I would share little snippets of my experience as well as the tidal wave of emotions that flooded my body when I would start to talk. I would try to find the words but would quickly become overwhelmed and unable to make sense of what to say next. With this pressure and strain, I decided that talking about this felt emotionally dangerous for me and I would lock up and turn inwards.

This changed in 2014 when I visited a sand therapist to explore burnout and fatigue.

I didn't think that I would be talking about my history as a survivor at all, and yet within the first session, I was crying my heart out while protecting a little symbol in a sand tray that represented my eight-year-old self. I had not realized what was happening as I began to build my life in that tray that day. I chose symbols to represent family members and loved ones and a little glass rainbow to represent lost pets who had crossed the rainbow bridge. I chose symbols to represent significant relationships in my world and then I chose this black messy-looking shiny rock to sit in the corner of the tray.

As we began to explore the tray, I felt constantly pulled towards this black rock but didn't want to investigate what this could mean for me because something was feeling uncomfortable inside and I still had no conscious idea of what this feeling was about.

After half a session spent exploring all these other symbols, I was left with just the one. At this point, I felt physically sick to my stomach and began to feel very ungrounded and shaky. I felt an overwhelming tornado of emotions beginning to work their way from the pit of my stomach and up through my throat. I felt the need to cry so hard that my face hurt. I felt such a deep sense of hurt and anger and confusion that I couldn't speak at all, and I sobbed for what felt like hours but only lasted seconds. As I was able to reground and reconnect with my tray, I noticed that I had been cradling the symbol that represented me. A little bright heart in the centre of the tray and suddenly a lightning vision struck me with such significance that I can still remember holding my breath and waiting for the roof to collapse on me. It was now obvious why I was cradling this little heart. I needed it out of the tray and out of the line of sight of the threatening black stone in the corner – the dominating and overpowering presence of my perpetrator feeding off my emotions in the tray.

I was invited to say what I needed to say to this stone and to complete the tray in any way that felt good for me. I wrote the words 'no more' in the sand and removed him from the tray. The therapist supported me to throw the perpetrator out of the window and out of sight, and I chose at this point to give him no more power over my life. A decision that still empowers me today!

What this therapist did for me was to hold, nurture, nudge and empower me. This was the beginning of a newfound love for sand trays and symbols, and as I continued on my own journey of qualifying as a therapist and starting my own practice, this experience fuelled many decisions that I would come to make as I began to grow our Creative Counsellors Movement and develop this framework.

I love to have a framework to work within but when I qualified as an Integrative Counsellor and began to combine creative interventions in my work, there wasn't a framework anywhere to take inspiration from. I couldn't find any social media communities, diagrams or books written around Creative Counselling. There were plenty of inspiring books around Art Therapy approaches and sand-play techniques, but I was happy with my Integrative Counselling approach and I didn't want to have to retrain to lose the approach that I was convinced could be complemented to support clients who hadn't yet been able to find the words to talk. So, over the years, I devised an approach that would work for me. As I began to share this with colleagues and friends within my therapy circles, they too found this useful. It is an ever-growing, ever-evolving concept, which I believe, like everything in the Creative Counselling approach, will grow, adapt, change and become a thriving model in the Creative Counsellors Community.

THE CREATE CIRCLE APPROACH

We will explore the Create Circle Approach throughout this book, but it is helpful to give a brief introduction to this model, as it is the seed from which all the book's chapters find their roots.

When I sat down to design this Create Circle, I thought about all the elements that help to strengthen our Creative Counselling approach so we can support clients as well as ourselves during the counselling work. During this process, I fell in love with the idea of therapy being like a dance between two people. Sometimes a fiery tango, sometimes a gentle and nudging tap and sometimes a dramatic ballet. If we think of the therapy process as a dance, I believe that a thriving Creative Counsellor finds ways to balance both the client's needs and the needs of the counsellor in the room. Both the client and the counsellor will find times when they need to take the lead, and both need guidance, nurture and support to transform and grow.

I hope that this model inspires you to find balance and empowers you to create beautiful, nurturing and transformational spaces for both you and your client.

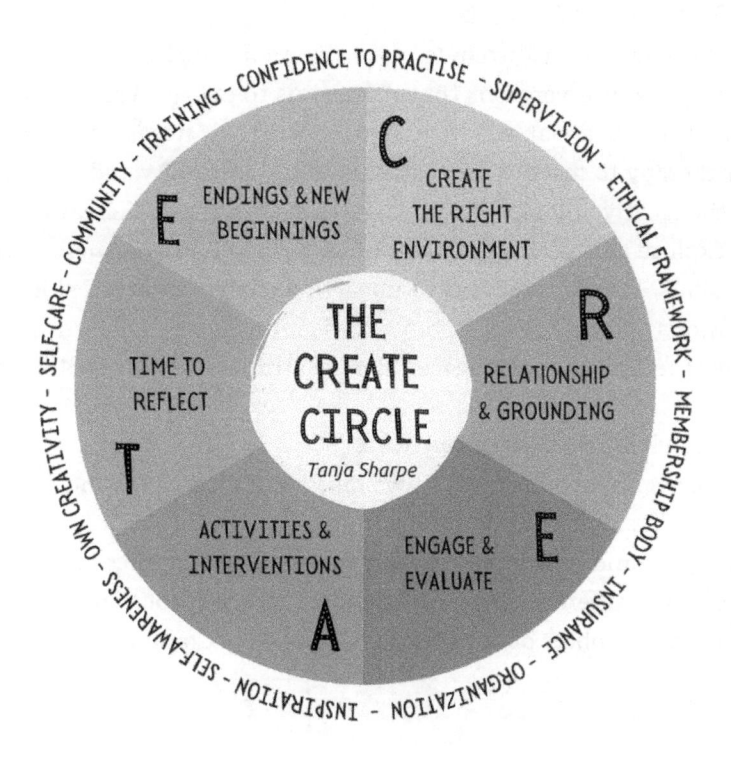

THE CREATE CIRCLE
Tanja Sharpe

- **C** — CREATE THE RIGHT ENVIRONMENT
- **R** — RELATIONSHIP & GROUNDING
- **E** — ENGAGE & EVALUATE
- **A** — ACTIVITIES & INTERVENTIONS
- **T** — TIME TO REFLECT
- **E** — ENDINGS & NEW BEGINNINGS

Outer ring: TRAINING – CONFIDENCE TO PRACTISE – SUPERVISION – ETHICAL FRAMEWORK – MEMBERSHIP BODY – INSURANCE – ORGANIZATION – INSPIRATION – SELF-AWARENESS – OWN CREATIVITY – SELF-CARE – COMMUNITY

1. Create the Right Environment

In this element of the circle, I explore how to create a nurturing, creative and curious environment in which the client and therapist can ground, grow and blossom together – from setting up your room, to choosing symbols, to working online or outside. We will explore how creating the right environment is the foundation of the Creative Counselling relationship, just as a tree begins to grow from the soil.

2. Relationship and Grounding

In this element of the circle, I explore how we creatively nurture the therapeutic relationship and alliance as well as the importance of grounding in Creative Counselling work to facilitate a safe working environment for both the client and the therapist. This is an important part of the work that means clients feel included in the process of therapy and empowered to make choices for themselves that meet their needs. Just as a tree needs certain conditions to grow and thrive, we too need certain conditions in the creative space.

3. Engage and Evaluate

In this element of the circle, we navigate our way through a range of creative interventions that support us to engage with and assess where clients are at and how to prioritize their needs and set goals for therapy to foster a sense of shared responsibility and autonomy in the creative therapeutic process. I guide us through creative ways to explore goal setting, evaluation and ongoing assessment within sessions. We explore ways to unearth a client's interest, skills and passions and how to incorporate these into the creative work so that clients feel connected, engaged and held throughout the relationship.

4. Activities and Interventions

In this element of the circle, we discover new playful and creative ways to facilitate interventions that help clients to process difficult emotions and create new insight into their experiences of life. We work with different methods, concepts, interventions and tools and welcome members of our Creative Counsellors Community to join us and share some of their inspiring and favourite creative interventions in the counselling room.

5. Time to Reflect
In this element of the circle, we explore how important it is to facilitate a time to process and reflect on any learning and awareness gained within the Creative Counselling process. I will introduce some examples of ways to reflect creatively on the work and to engage with clients in the process.

6. Endings and New Beginnings
In this element of the approach, I explore the importance of endings and how every ending actually starts at the beginning. We explore creative ways to navigate and celebrate the final stage in the process and different types of endings that we may encounter in the therapy room.

7. Exploring the I in *CreatIvIty*
For our Create Circle Approach to thrive, we need strong, nurturing and supportive boundaries, and in this element of the circle, we explore all the other factors that support us to bring our most confident and creative selves to the therapy room.

While writing this book, I also thought it was important to share with you three core principles that I developed early on in my work and have held close to my heart while growing this approach.

1. To commit to **exploring** how, together, clients and counsellors can co-create safe and nurturing creative spaces.
2. To commit to **empowering** clients to move towards being autonomous and self-guiding while working creatively.
3. To **reflect** on the process of the work from a creative, heart-led and compassionate approach for both client and counsellor.

I am excited to see how these principles are taking root in the work that we are already doing and am curious to see how these will adapt and change within Creative Counselling culture in the future.

CAN CREATIVE INTERVENTIONS BE INTEGRATED INTO ANY CORE COUNSELLING MODEL?

I have yet to hear of a model that cannot be complemented by offering creative interventions! Many counsellors are already working creatively without even knowing it. Simply working with a piece of paper and some coloured pens is offering a form of creativity in which clients can make sense of their situation through lines, shapes and colours. I believe that creativity can be integrated into any counselling model, and we can see examples everywhere we look in the therapeutic world – from movement-based therapies, to talking therapies, to walking and talking while engaging with nature as a co-therapist. As we grow our Creative Counsellors Movement, we are connecting with more and more counsellors who are inviting clients to creatively explore different parts of themselves that they may otherwise have hidden away, and we are now seeing a shift towards training and ongoing professional development that offer these ways of working.

WHAT IF I AM NOT CREATIVE?

One of the biggest fears that I come across daily in my work is the belief that 'I am not creative'. This is often the impact of judgement and messages received in childhood. Many of us can relate to being told that the penguin we drew looks like a dinosaur or how we haven't coloured within the lines properly. Or never being chosen to win the Christmas card design competition or being singled out for being too 'outside the box' in art class when giving the apple a face and a name.

I remember when a teacher told me that I was a daydreamer and that it showed in my art. That daydreamers don't get jobs and I would never go anywhere in life if I didn't stop staring out of the window and drawing little pixies in mushroom houses. She was so full of judgement and would encourage the whole class to laugh at and learn from my mistakes. She would make me sit and draw a bowl full of apples and bananas, and when I wanted to give my banana some wings so that it could fly to banana land and make new friends, I would be scolded and would have to start all over again. My imagination became a problem at school, so I began to turn away from my creative spark in an attempt to fit in and not be singled out all the time. Oh, how I wish I could go back and let my eight-year-old self know that in the future I would build a career out of helping others to be creative, writing 'doodling books' and expressing my most creative self in my work and my life.

As we integrate these painful experiences around 'not being creative', it can be easy to forget how intrinsically creative we actually are as human beings. In essence, every part of life is a creative process.

We are all being creative in every way in every day. We create the meals that we like to eat, often choosing ingredients that smell good and presenting our food in a way that looks good on the plate. We choose the clothes that we wear, often opting for colours and fabrics that represent our moods and how we feel on the day. We are often expressing ourselves through make up, hair, clothing and colour. When we are walking in nature, we might stop to take in the beautiful colours of the sunrise and sunsets. We tune in to the sounds of the ocean as the waves crash onto the shore and watch as seagulls swoop down and move playfully together in the clouds. We look for patterns and shapes everywhere we go, appreciating the unique shapes that frost creates on a window or spiderwebs in the garden. We appreciate beautiful art, and during celebratory times of the year, we decorate our homes with colour, symbols and metaphor. We choose what furniture and colour schemes we are drawn to in our homes and we often find that different colours create different feelings within us.

> **PRACTICE:** Take a moment to tune in to your creative process where you are now. What colours are you wearing? What surrounds you? What images, patterns and shapes can you see?

WHY CREATIVE COUNSELLING NOW?

In 2018, I was chosen alongside 114 other community leaders from 46 different countries to represent our Creative Counsellors Global Movement in the Facebook Community Leadership Program. This was in recognition of our dedication to growing a community that creates change and is inspiring impact in the world. Landing in San Francisco, I met the most incredible human, Suzanne Alderson, who has become family to me and has become an advocate for and supported the Creative Counsellors Movement since.

Suzanne founded Parenting Mental Health, a global community dedicated to *ending generational mental illness* and supporting parents/carers of children who struggle with their mental health. Together, we navigated our time in the programme and met with other community leaders, many of whom shared with us a similar story: that wherever they were in the world, people's mental health was suffering. I spent time with community leaders whose missions and communities were dedicated to supporting refugees of war, to supporting women to leave violent relationships, to helping young people who are victims of trafficking and to supporting economically disadvantaged families to survive and thrive. I talked with young people challenging gun laws who had survived school shootings, and I spent time with other leaders who wanted to know about the differences in mental health support in the UK and Africa.

I sat around the fire with incredible leaders who shared their mental health stories that fuelled the birth of their communities, like Mel Bound, who founded This Mum Runs, the world's largest running community for women after suffering a miscarriage and battled with depression, and Dave Cornthwaite, the founder of YesTribe, who beat depression by adventuring through the world in nature. We are surrounded by inspiring stories of outside-the-box ways that people are finding to navigate their mental health struggles, and I believe that we can take some inspiration from this to breathe new life into our therapy approaches.

As a proactive counsellor involved in many social media groups, I see so many clients sharing their experiences of therapy. Many clients share stories about being told that 'they are not ready' or 'the approach is not right for them' or even worse, being told that 'they don't engage' and having to leave. I have heard stories of clients who have been sitting on six-month waiting lists finally stepping through the door, being asked 'So, what would you like to talk about today?' and not knowing where to start or what to say. I hear of clients who believe that 'therapy doesn't work for them' and others going in and out of therapy services for a lifetime because they have never really been able to work with the core of their issues, feelings, experiences and emotions, as the words to express their story haven't been invented.

In a press release of 5 March 2021, the UK's Department of Health and Social Care announced that recent NHS research suggested that one in six young people were struggling with a mental health problem, a rise from 2017 when the figure was one in nine (Department of Health and Social Care 2021). I would suggest that these are the cases we know about and that the figures are potentially even worse. The UK Office for National Statistics (2021) shared that between 27 January and 7 March 2021, one in five adults reported experiencing some form of depression, an increase of 19 per cent from the year before. As a global community, we are facing the threat of the COVID-19 pandemic, ever-growing financial struggles, increased mental health challenges and mental health services that are struggling to meet the demand of those who need them most. I hear from clients who are desperate for help as a result of being on waiting lists for more than a year, and in some cases even up to three years, for complex mental health issues.

We are in the midst of a global mental health storm that is having a devastating impact on people's mental health and capsizing the hopes for a healthy future for many clients. Couple this with a growing need for more expressive ways to empower clients to express their stories and we have identified a global need for a new, brave and courageous kind of counsellor. The kind of counsellor who will offer nurturing creative interventions to facilitate spaces for clients who have felt like a square peg in a round hole after not 'fitting into the box' that they have been met with when entering a therapy service. The research, coupled with my own experience, is showing us that what we are doing is important and it makes a difference.

So, why Creative Counselling now? Why on earth not?

Chapter 2

Create the Right Environment

This is the first element of our Create Circle Approach and helps us to consider what each client may need from a therapeutic environment to help them to thrive within the space. In my experience, environments do have an impact on the client's ability to engage, and if we are to truly respect the client's autonomy, it can be helpful to think about how we can create flexible and adaptive spaces to meet our clients where they are at.

EXPLORING DIFFERENT CREATIVE COUNSELLING ENVIRONMENTS

> **PRACTICE:** Take a moment right now to think about what environment you feel most calm in. Is it tucked away on your sofa with a book? Is it walking through the forest on a sunny day? Is it watching the waves crashing on the shoreline? Is it playing a favourite game online with friends?

One of the skills that we have as Creative Counsellors is to be able to travel with clients through their different lenses and worlds to meet them where they are at. This often involves switching environments and creating unique spaces that feel individually suited to the needs of each client.

We know that clients need different things from therapy, and this includes the environment. Think of this as a unique part of the process and an important one. What does your client need most? Would your client feel more at ease amongst the trees in the sunshine? Or would they feel safer indoors? I have witnessed incredible shifts in the relationship and energy when I have invited clients to decide where the therapy will take place – offering a new perspective, promoting autonomy and creating a balance in the power dynamics in the relationship.

Matching the client with the right environment enables clients to heal in their own way and at their own pace. I think back to when I was a teen and remember just how important the beach was to me in my recovery from post-traumatic stress disorder (PTSD). I can imagine how powerful it would have been to have received therapy in the place where I felt most at home. My own healing sanctuary. To have had the space to write poetry in the sand and have someone to share this with. The minute I stepped into a therapy room and sat on a sofa opposite a psychologist, I just froze up. This did not feel right. I did not feel in control of this situation. I was not able to be myself there and I was well out of my window of tolerance. My emotional state was disconnected, and therapy in this environment was never going to work for me. I can now see that this environment mirrored the traumatic experiences that I had been through in interview rooms with the police and other professionals who were trying to help at the time. Everyone wanting and expecting me to talk and to have the right words for them. No one understanding that I wasn't ready. Pushing and pulling and forcing some kind of reaction from me.

Had someone invited a walk on the beach and a space to breathe that open air, I believe I would have been able to form a therapeutic relationship and I would have been able to tell my story.

We can facilitate transformational spaces indoors, outdoors, in forests, in parks, on the phone, virtually through video calls, in the client's home, at school and in the workplace, to name just a few. We can empower clients to make choices that feel right for them and feel safe and okay for us to facilitate. A space to be, to heal and to transform.

> **KEY POINT:** Different environments speak to different clients. What does your client most need?

INDOOR THERAPY ROOMS

I remember how excited I was to turn the key and open the door to my first ever therapy room. It was a blank space. White walls and blue dotted carpets. It was a small room with plenty of light coming through the windows; however, it didn't have a view of the outside. I looked into the hallway of a clinical-looking business centre, and I didn't know then that this would spark an interest in understanding how the environment impacts on the quality of the therapy.

So, as I started to turn this blank slate into my version of an Aladdin's Cave full of creative treasures to explore, I was optimistic about what was to come. I created a chalkboard wall for expressing emotions and experiences through doodling. I built a sand tray to fit the unique shape of the room, and I discovered that I could find little hiding places for symbols and miniatures everywhere. I hung different nets from the walls to house puppets and colourful stuffed animals, and I filled boxes with clay and playdough for messy play. I was determined to create a healing space for all the young people that I was going to be working with.

When I opened my doors, the real adventure began.

> **PRACTICE:** Take a moment to experience your Creative Counselling space through the eyes of a client. What journey do they take on arriving? What do they see? What is the lighting like and is it adjustable? What colours have you chosen for your environment and how might this impact on the client? What else do you notice? Do you ever invite feedback from clients on the space? Could this be helpful?

NEURODIVERSITY AND ROOM LIGHTING

I supported many autistic young people and their families and through this I learned the importance of getting the lighting right. The room had standard office fluorescent lighting, and this was often very annoying for my clients and manifested physically in different ways – from headaches, to nausea, to anxiety. I replaced this lighting with different styles of lamps in each of corner of the room, and clients would ask for different lamps to be turned on and off. I ended up rehoming many lamps and lights over the years to make way for dimmable lights that could be adjusted to suit my clients' sensory needs. Adding lava lamps and mood lighting formed an important part of the therapy process. 'What colour would you like to choose today and why?'

Since moving from this room to a space with big open windows and views into the outdoors, I notice how much more transforming this is for clients. There is something very calming and in tune with the rhythms of our own bodies about seeing nature and natural light. I still have dimmable lighting and various sensory-based colour lighting but the need for this has changed, as clients often prefer natural lighting to anything synthetic. I think this makes sense. We are products of nature and our bodies have always been in tune with the light that nature provides.

> **KEY POINT:** Adjusting the lighting in the room can have a real impact on the client's ability to be present, to feel safe and to feel connected.

SOURCING RESOURCES FOR YOUR THERAPY ROOM

Searching for new resources can easily become an expensive hobby, and I am always on the lookout. I love to wander through car-boot sales and second-hand shops looking for treasures that clients can relate to. A string of pearls, an old glass perfume bottle, a set of small woodland fairies, a chipped little heart or a ceramic dog. All these incredible metaphors and symbols can create an emotional connection for clients and become the transformational tool that helps them to bridge the unconscious with the conscious so it can be worked with. To enable clients to tell their story, we need a diverse range of resources that represent different life situations. However, if you are starting out, it's important to know that you are already creative and can support clients' creativity simply with a pen and paper. I have been building my creative collection for years and will always keep searching for new and exciting tools for my therapy room. So, start with what you have and build at a pace that feels good for you. Here are some suggestions.

- A variety of paper, card, journals and other writing materials for clients to use. This is great for doodling, free-writing activities, collage work and art.
- Coloured pens, felt tips, pencils and pens.
- A sand container or tray. When you are getting started, the trays that you buy will often depend on the size of your room and your budget. You can also find inflatable sand containers and could even use cat-litter trays, which are portable and easy to have with you in the boot of your car if need be. I am lucky to have a sand-tray designer in the family and have a selection of trays in varying sizes, shapes and designs, from hexagonal trays for creating beautiful 'sandalas' (mandalas in the sand) to full-size trays. You will also need to source good-quality play sand that is non-toxic to touch. You can often purchase this from toy stores and supermarkets. Sand often arrives damp, so you will need to dry it out in your tray before using it. This can take up to a week depending on the environment. I usually add enough sand to fill half the tray.
- A range of different symbols to work with, including people who represent family members like grandad, mother, baby, child, father, brother, etc.; emergency workers, doctors and social workers; teachers and sportspeople.
- Fairy-tale symbols that represent goblins, pirates, mermaids, princesses, princes, kings, queens, dragons, fairies, witches and wizards.
- Soldiers and symbols that represent war and conflict.
- Religious and spiritual symbols representing as many faiths as possible, including angels, deities, priests, nuns, Buddhas, Hindi symbols, crosses, Islamic symbols, Christian symbols and Catholic symbols. Chalice well and the golden cup.
- Historic and cultural symbols, including Egyptian, African, Jamaican, Aboriginal and British, to name just a few.
- Comic, cartoon, movie and superhero symbols, including Batman, Superwoman, Spider-Man, Ninja Turtles, Scooby-Doo, Lord of the Rings figures and Daleks.
- Symbols that represent end of life, such as tunnels, skulls, coffins, skeletons, gravestones, bare trees and angels.

- Natural symbols collected on walks, like leaves, dried flowers, sticks, stones, moss and bark. Remember to leave a positive footprint in nature, not disturbing the ecosystem or damaging the environment as you collect.
- Transport symbols, like cars, boats, trucks, tanks, planes, space rockets, helicopters, traffic lights, stop signs and road signs.
- Bridges and fences – think of boundaries and connectors. Many powerful conversations with clients have been inspired simply by placing a bridge in the sand. I have sourced some great ones from fish tank suppliers – they are often the perfect size.
- Jenga pieces and wooden blocks to create height. Stone walls and other 'building'-type symbols.
- Crystals, rocks and stones.
- Rainbows, sunshine and moon-shaped symbols.
- Pets, animals and mythical creatures.
- Symbols that represent wheelchairs and other abilities and disabilities.
- A variety of house symbols, like chairs, beds and other furniture.
- Symbols that represent a rainbow of colours in the room.
- Angry symbols, like the two-headed dog or the growling fire-breathing dragon.
- Symbols that represent other emotions and feelings.
- Puppets and paper bags to create personalized puppets.
- Scarves, material, dress-up costumes, hats, gloves, etc. for role play.
- Cards for working with, such as emotion cards and certain oracle sets. It's important to work with these yourself first, as some cards can be dangerous in the therapeutic space. Avoid stocking cards that have an aspect of 'telling your future', as these can cause a rupture in the therapeutic relationship and foster a 'fixing' kind of thinking. Clients will often bring their own cards into the room, which is really powerful to work with.
- Images and photos. I print and laminate images and photos that I have taken or found on royalty-free sites. These are powerful aids in helping clients to connect with their feelings, emotions and experiences.
- Colouring, sketch or doodle books.

- Paints, watercolours, acrylics and paintbrushes.
- Glue, anything that sparkles and can be added such as lace, ribbon, washi tape, etc.
- Magazines for ripping up and adding layers and texture to collage work.

There are plenty of places to find creative resources, including toy shops, supermarkets, car-boot sales, charity shops, social media 'for-sale' sites, groups and garden centres. Reaching out to friends and family can also be helpful, as they will often keep an eye out for symbols and resources for you.

> **KEY POINT:** Clients will respond differently to different tools and symbols. Work towards having a range of creative tools and symbols that can be used to represent different emotions, life stages, beliefs, interests, genders, values, cultures, life experiences and abilities. Without this, you run the risk of resourcing for the few instead of the many.

CREATING DIVERSE THERAPY SPACES

PRACTICE: Take a moment to explore the following questions. What does diversity and culture mean to you? How inclusive is your space, really? What more can you do?

When I first set up my therapy room, I thought that I was doing the best that I could to represent different genders, sexualities, ages and beliefs. What I didn't consider deeply at the time was that I lacked representation of cultural diversity by not representing all the skin tones, cultures, heritages and spiritualities in our wonderful world. I stocked books filled with white princesses and white emergency workers in suits. I look back now and remember that many if not all of my books featured white faces and stereotypes. How traumatizing and disempowering this could have been for clients who were underrepresented in my therapy space.

I have seen the impact of racial inequality both as a child growing up in South Africa and in the experiences that my son has faced in his lifetime. My son is of mixed heritage, and he was often the only child of any other colour but white in his class. He now describes his experiences of growing up in the UK as 'feeling like an alien'. Many if not all of his reading lists and schoolbooks were written by white authors, and he doesn't remember having a teacher who wasn't white. Growing up as a mixed-heritage, autistic boy, he faced many overlapping systems and experiences of discrimination and disadvantage. This idea of being different and the confusion around this was triggered even more when he stepped into a therapy room at age nine with a white therapist who, with good intentions, tried to convince him that the other children didn't think that he was different or 'an alien'. He felt one thing but was being told something else. He couldn't make sense of this at the time; it was disempowering, and it invalidated his experiences and feelings.

We have a responsibility and a duty to create inclusive, diverse and culturally represented therapy spaces. It's important that when we begin to build our resources, we consider this in what we stock and how we display our materials.

We are now finally beginning to see more culturally diverse resources being created and shared, and it is becoming easier to find these. From colouring books representing African heritage, to symbols that feature Hindu celebrations and everything in between. Think about any art that you have on your walls and the books that you stock on your shelves. Think about your website and social media channels. Consider how you can be advocating for creative and inclusive therapeutic spaces before the client even makes contact. Then consider the journey that a client will take on entering your space. What will they see and what might they feel?

> **KEY POINT:** It's important to create diverse and inclusive spaces that celebrate culture, heritage and individual experience.

STORING RESOURCES IN YOUR THERAPY ROOM

Many Creative Counsellors can identify with the challenges that come with trying to find enough space to house all the resources in our therapy room, especially as many of us are always on the lookout for new, quirky, emotive and unique tools that could help clients to share their stories with us. I am always looking! My partner knows that when we travel anywhere or take a walk, I am on the lookout for that extra something for my kit.

Last year, my partner and I spent ten days exploring the Scottish Highlands in Jasper, our quirky converted campervan. We found ourselves off-grid in some of the most wild and beautiful places, and in most if not all of these places, I found little trinkets, symbols and gifts that can be used in the sand tray and creatively in the counselling room.

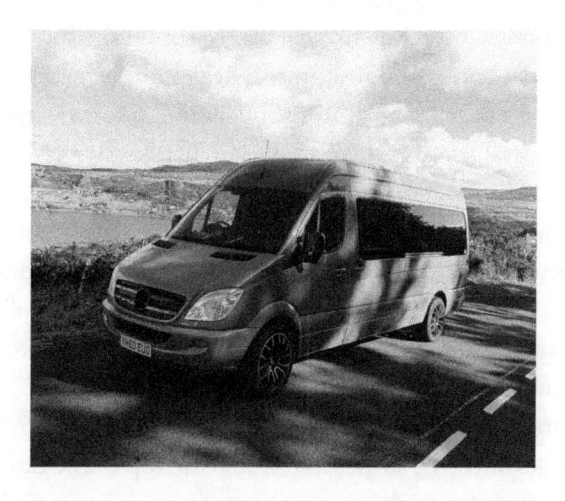

During one of our daily adventures, I found myself at Cast Off Crafts, a treasure trove of upcycled and recycled trinkets and goods.

We were met by Shuggie the springer spaniel, who never left our sides as we explored the shop. The shop was filled with symbols and creative materials that could be utilized in the therapy space, like painted stones, sea-glass symbols, hand-knitted puppets, photos and images of beautiful scenery and storybooks. Everything had been handmade locally with the help of local artists.

I left that day with some hand-sewn tie-dyed fish, driftwood symbols, finger puppets and a friend for life in Shuggie. We also learned about many of the local stories from the owner, including where we needed to visit next to see the puffins. The puffins even made their way into my therapy room as part of my images collection for clients to explore their emotions by working with aspects of animals. Many counsellors in our Facebook group share the symbols that they collect for their counselling toolbox while they're out and about, and this has become a talking point in our community.

So, now that we are collecting all these wonderful resources, how do we store them? I get asked this all the time, and I am going to share the ways that work best for me.

My room is set up so that all the activities take place around the edges of the room and our seating area is in the centre. This way, I feel like I can create a space for clients to begin and end sessions in the same place, which feels grounding and safe.

I have simple white Ikea storage units around the room that house all the symbols, books and resources, with enough space to explore in between. I use a coat stand to store any puppets, scarves and material, which works well as it is tall and takes up little space.

I have a decent-sized six-foot folding table that sits just under the main window at the edge of the room, and this is where we create art together. On the table, I store paintbrushes, paints, water pots and other useful items that I work with. I also have small units with pull-out drawers on the table, which store smaller art items, like glitter, jewels and glue.

In the centre of the room, I have a round coffee table with storage areas underneath, and this means that I can store bowls of extra resources, like buttons, stones and wool. The top of the table becomes our sand-tray area, which is a great way to encourage exploration of the room around the tray for resources.

On one side of the room, I have an abundance of plant life that provides a place to explore little ecosystems and can house clay creations while they are drying. These also double as interesting icebreaker conversation starters to help clients talk about self-care, nurture, nourishment and growth. When the leaves fall, this helps us to explore sensitive topics around endings, beginnings and death, which can be held beautifully in creative work.

Some counsellors like to colour code their creative spaces. I found myself in awe of fellow Creative Counsellor Masha Bennett's room in Glossop when I visited in 2021 to attend an Integrative Sandplay training. As I opened the door to her room, I was met with crisp, white walls and a sea of expressive, colourful and playful symbols from wall to wall. She had colour coded her symbols in some spaces so you could be drawn to working with colour, which I found really appealing during our training. I felt drawn to the greens and golds when thinking about my spiritual self. I was drawn to pinks and purples for healing and to nurturing shades of teal and blue when exploring my creative self. I felt empowered to make choices that suited my needs in the moment and the space held me beautifully to do just that!

There are so many ways that we can set up our rooms as therapists, and this diversity is what we love to celebrate in our Creative Counsellors Community!

On entering my room, you will be met with orange and white walls with plenty of balancing greenery. As there is so much colour around us, I aim to balance this with a simple white storage theme that reduces sensory stimulation, which can sometimes feel overwhelming for clients. I have found that some clients need a very calm environment and respond well to being introduced to resources at a gentler pace over time. In my experience, this is especially true for clients who have experienced childhood trauma, as being faced by many resources that appear playful can often induce a sense of fear or trigger an overwhelming anxiety response. I find that covering certain aspects of the storage units with a light fabric (that can be tied back) can reduce anxiety for clients who struggle with this way of working.

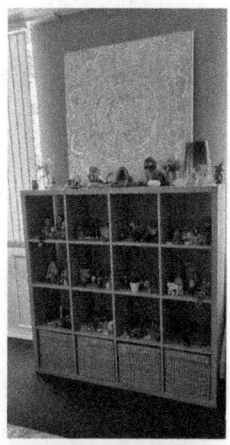

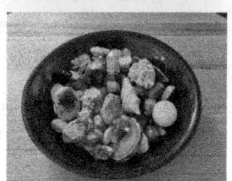

Even though you may find that some clients struggle with lots of stimulation, many clients love to be able to arrive in an Aladdin's Cave and be met with a playful, stimulating and creative environment. As you develop your creative practice, you will get to know each client and their individual needs. This will empower you to be able to adjust your room in ways that support your clients' autonomy and meet their needs too.

CARRYING RESOURCES AS A MOBILE COUNSELLOR

We have explored how to set up your counselling room, but what if you are a mobile therapist and on the go? For many years, I would meet clients in their homes or travel between schools and practices, and I needed to develop a way of offering a range of resources on the move. There are a few hints and tips that I have found along the way that I would like to share with you.

- Laminating photos of your symbols is a great way build your collection without needing the space to physically house them. They take up very little room when being transported, and this enables you to work with symbols and metaphors in portable sand trays.
- Keep sand in a plastic bag that is sized to fit your sand tray. I take clear plastic bags and cut them to size to fit my sand tray. I store the sand in the bag and tie it up; when setting up for clients, I untie the bag and neatly store the sand and the bag together in the tray.
- Some sand trays have lids and are much more portable. I have a hexagonal sand tray that is a client favourite due to the shape. This comes with a lid, which I secure with big ties when it's not in use, and I keep the sand in the tray. You can also use inflatable sand trays or cat-litter boxes, as these are very transportable.
- Digital resources are also available and we are seeing more and more of these being developed. A tablet or laptop can be a handy resource for this. If you search for 'digital therapy resources' online, you will find a range of interesting ways of working.
- Art can also be worked with digitally, and there are apps that support this. If you need to travel and prefer a hands-on approach, which I most definitely do, you can find some great art travel bags in your local art supplies stores and online. Beauty travel kits and bags work well too, as they have many little secret storage solutions to help you.

As Creative Counselling grows, I predict that we will see many new products come to life to solve our storage troubles!

VIRTUAL COUNSELLING – WORKING CREATIVELY ONLINE

We have seen huge growth in the area of virtual counselling in light of the COVID-19 pandemic, and there are some questions around how to work creatively online, which can feel different for clients and therapists alike.

I want to share my own experience of this, and although there is little written about this topic, I hope to inspire you to know that creativity can happen in any space, including a virtual environment.

During 2020, my team and I developed and delivered a programme titled '40 Ways to Work Creatively Online' within our Creative Counsellors CPD Membership. This proved to be very popular and we soon found that other counsellors began to offer similar trainings. We knew then that we were starting to see an exciting shift in confidence around delivering these interventions online.

We learned many things in taking our practices online, including which exercises flowed with ease and which needed tweaking and adjusting to suit our clients and their presenting issues. One thing that I am sure of is that online working can be more tiring. Many therapists in our community share this viewpoint, and conversations around 'always being online', 'the boundaries feeling different' and 'sitting for so much of the day' have dominated our discussions. Because of the impact that this can have on our own emotional and physical wellbeing as counsellors, it is important to recognize any increased needs for self-care so that we can reflect, adapt and change how we take care of ourselves when not working. I have found that I often feel as though I have been drained of energy at the end of a long day online and spending more time in nature re-energizes and balances me.

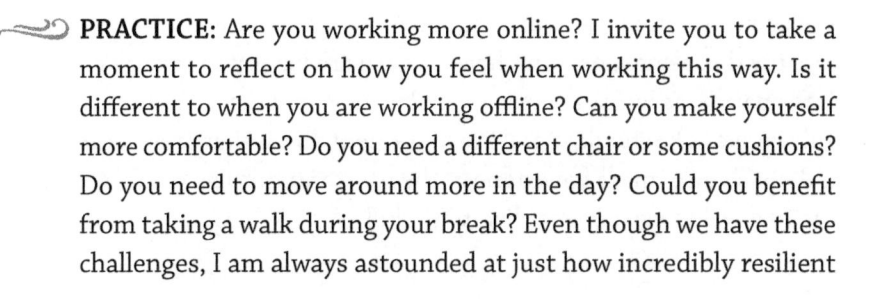

> **PRACTICE:** Are you working more online? I invite you to take a moment to reflect on how you feel when working this way. Is it different to when you are working offline? Can you make yourself more comfortable? Do you need a different chair or some cushions? Do you need to move around more in the day? Could you benefit from taking a walk during your break? Even though we have these challenges, I am always astounded at just how incredibly resilient

and Creative Counsellors are in adapting to new situations and environments while sharing ideas and offering support to others.

There are some very important aspects to be aware of while working online. There are issues around technology and changes in the therapy relationship and dynamic, as well as confidentiality and privacy to be aware of.

Some clients have voiced that working online from their homes during lockdown has been a challenge for many reasons, including fear of being overheard, being interrupted by family members, not having space to be able to process emotions after sessions such as working out at the gym and feeling like the therapist is in their home, nest or space.

The British Association for Counselling and Psychotherapy (BACP) ordinarily recommends lengthy training to practise as an online counsellor, however they have recognized the need for counsellors to be able to continue to support the mental health of their clients in extreme circumstances and we have seen a growth in organizations offering online training for counsellors. As counsellors have found themselves thrown in at the deep end in many situations, we have seen creativity thrive and, as such, skills are growing in this area.

In this section, we will explore some of the common myths, facts and points to consider when working online with clients.

Body Language

When we are working in a room with clients, we are able to take in the whole person and how they present in the space for us. We are reading cues from top to toe and feeling energy shifts in the space. We can also see how they creatively interact with the space around them, and this gives us many clues as to how to proceed, shift, change and support the client. In an online world, this can feel quite different in that we are mostly seeing a person's head and we are having to take as much information as we can about what else may be happening from very subtle clues like shoulder and eye movement. I find that I rely more on a client's voice than I have done in the past, and this has really helped me to develop even deeper listening skills.

Working at Depth

There have been questions around whether clients and therapists can work as deeply in an online environment and whether relational depth is negatively impacted. I can assure you from my own experience, and that of many therapists working in this way, that this has not been the experience for many. In fact, we are seeing an increase in how many clients are positively impacted by offering an online therapeutic relationship. Many clients who have struggled to access therapy in the past are reporting that being able to access therapy from the privacy of their own homes and their 'safe spaces' has enabled them to build therapeutic trust, which in turn has supported working at relational depth in an online environment. Aisling Treanor described in her research that 'five out of seven participants shared that relational depth could be experienced in online therapy' and that participants described the experience as 'unforgettable, beyond words and life changing' (Treanor 2017).

Online Counselling Is Not For Everyone

For some clients, online working is absolutely not appropriate, and we have to be able to assess the needs of clients and be transparent and congruent in what we can safely facilitate. I know that for many clients who are surviving domestic violence or who have issues around their marriage and relationships, online working has not been an option. On occasion, clients and therapists are sharing that online counselling just isn't working, and this is individual to each client.

Technology

For some counsellors and clients, the world of technology has been too overwhelming to navigate, and this needs to be considered when making the choice to move online. This has been particularly challenging for some of our elderly communities, who have reported that online working was not an option for them. We also must consider that some clients and therapists have not had the financial means to invest in the technology needed to access online services, and many rely on the help of others, such as younger people, to ensure that they can connect in a virtual world. We need to consider technology and how we may support clients who would like to access support but need a little extra help to do so.

Therapist Confidence in Holding the Space

It can take some time to become confident in facilitating counselling online with the many technical and 'in-the-moment' challenges that can present without warning, such as a poor Wi-Fi connection or a headset not working. With boundaries being an essential part of the therapeutic process, you may find that during a session a client's dog is constantly interrupting and needing to be removed from the room or the doorbell keeps ringing, and this can be exhausting to manage at times. Talking through any possible challenges that clients may face during the contracting and assessment phase can be helpful in understanding how best to support clients and maintain your boundaries. Having a backup plan in case technology throws you a curveball is essential, and the BACP has now included this in the *Ethical Framework for the Counselling Professions*. Knowing how you will contact your client if your online session is interrupted is an essential part of the work.

Confidentiality and Privacy

Using an encrypted service such as Zoom is important to maintain confidentiality for both you and your client. Ensuring that clients cannot record sessions without permission and going through all your sessions to ensure that you are working safely and ethically is important. I remember when I first started using Zoom, I shared my link with a friend to join me on a call. While we were catching up, I heard another voice and as if by magic another friend joined us on the same call. Since then, I have always ensured that the password feature is enabled and that all meetings have a unique ID. We must be aware that as we are working in people's private spaces, there may be others present in the space, sometimes without us even knowing. Exploring these topics in your contracting is important. I recommend that clients use headphones and check that they have a private space to be where they will not be overheard or interrupted. I am honest and I make it clear that I am unable to assure them of confidentiality in their space and that there is a shared responsibility around privacy for us to work together.

Set-Up

Consider the set-up of your space when working online. I have found that having a really comfortable chair with adjustable height can help, as well as having a wired internet connection where possible to avoid disconnection. I have creative resources to hand in case a client would like some support to be creative. I work with two cameras: one to focus on myself and another to attach to an overhead tripod to make it possible to share any creative resources and work. This is particularly helpful when I am receiving or facilitating Creative Supervision. I am mindful of the lighting in my room so that I appear in my true form to clients. I consider aspects like whether there is a window behind me, which can alter the light, or whether I am in a darkened space, which means clients struggle to see me.

Insurance

Before working online, it is vital that you check that you are insured. Get in touch with your insurance provider to clarify how you are working, what your individual policy is and how it applies to your work.

Supervision

It is helpful to work with a supervisor who has experience of working online and who can support you in your work. This work can feel different, and having someone who understands what this is like is an important way to nurture your confidence to practise.

Any Other Legal and Ethical Requirements to Practise

As this is an emerging field, there are many changes happening all the time that therapists need to be aware of as they navigate the online world. For instance, we need to be registered with the Information Commissioner's Office (ICO) and we need to ensure that any online platform that we work with is Health Insurance Portability and Accountability Act (HIPAA) compliant. If in doubt, always check it out!

With all these changes going on, how creative can we actually be? My answer to this is: as creative as you would like to be! I will share some of the ways that you can adapt your exercises and your practice to work with clients online from a creative perspective.

Visualization and Creative Mindfulness

This offers us a way to work with clients to ground and nurture themselves in an online space. We can invite clients to place their feet on the ground and breathe into their feet, focusing on how it feels to sit in the chair and recognize the steadiness of the ground. We can invite clients to visualize themselves in a safe space and to explore this with free writing or describing where this place is, what it is like and who may be there with them. We can invite clients to count as they breathe from one to ten and to envision a colour that they would like to work with to help them to explore a certain aspect of life, such as working with grief, pain, sexual violence, self-care, burnout, anxiety or the many other presenting issues clients bring into the therapy room.

Art

We can help clients to prepare for sessions during the contracting phase by exploring different creative interventions that they may like to work with. This way, we can empower clients to stock up on the items that they are drawn to engaging with in sessions. Think about how powerful this is for clients, as they are choosing what resources to have with them. In its simplest form, you can create art with a pen and some paper! You can invite clients to draw themselves in relation to their fears. How big are they compared with their fears and how do they present on paper? You can invite clients to draw an example of what they would like to explore during therapy and give their art a title or a voice. We will explore many creative interventions in Chapter 5 of this book!

Role Play

We can continue to offer interventions with puppets and role play by preparing clients for what they may like to have available for sessions. As puppets can be costly, we can invite clients to draw images on paper or paper bags and to work with these as we would in an in-person way. Many role-play activities don't require any extra resources, so these are great ways to support clients to work creatively and experientially online.

Collage
We can invite clients to print images, quotes and photos, as well as to collect magazines to create collage work. We can support clients to verbalize their thoughts and emotions and continue to hold the space as they create.

Working with Stories and Fairy Tales
We can help clients to write a dialogue between themselves and another character to explore a complicated relationship dynamic. Or even invite the client to create a story with themselves as the main character. What kind of character would you be and what is the storyline? Who else is in the story and where is it set?

Downloadable Resources
There are many downloadable resources available in our Creative Counsellors Membership Hub that can be used in your therapy space. You could add resources to the chat function in your chosen platform to help clients download and work with an intervention in real time.

These are just some examples of how you can adapt resources to support your practice!

> **PRACTICE:** Take a moment to think about all the resources that you have available to you and how you may adapt these for your online practice. What else could you consider? We share many ideas in our Facebook community, and you will be well supported by other members to build your creative toolbox there!

WORKING CREATIVELY IN THE OUTDOORS AND WALK-AND-TALK COUNSELLING
In Japan, there is a practice called 'Shinrin-Yoku', which translated into English means 'Forest Bath'. It is a practice that was developed in Japan during the 1980s, becoming a well-respected means of improving health and wellbeing in Japanese Medicine.

If you Google 'Shinrin-Yoku studies', you will find many articles about the health benefits of this practice and how 'spending time amongst the trees' has a positive impact on us. Simply put, spending time amongst the trees creates calming neuro-psychological effects that have a soothing response on the nervous system, reducing the stress hormone, cortisol, and supporting the immune system. In Japan, there are many beautiful stories and practices in which nature is the therapist.

Many of us turn to nature when we are looking to relax, express, make sense of our thoughts or emotions, wind down from a busy day, clear our minds or re-energize. We feel different amongst the trees, and nature offers us many metaphors that support our processing of complicated emotions and experiences. Like when we come across the tangled and stressed roots of a tree breaking through concrete to find a way to survive. Or how a snail retreats into its shell when it feels unsafe or in need of shelter from danger. We can utilize these healing elements and work with nature as a co-therapist to support our own self-care, while helping clients to process their thoughts and feelings, too. We can think of nature as our outdoor therapy room and as a safe container for our experiences.

It's no surprise that throughout the COVID-19 pandemic, many more counsellors began to express an interest in taking their counselling practice into the outdoors. Many new conversations were being sparked in our Creative Counsellors Community, and these conversations led to some beautifully inspiring and creative sharing sessions around outdoor practice. I was excited to see this develop, as I have always had a deep connection with nature and have experienced just how powerful an ally nature is as a therapeutic tool.

Before I qualified as a counsellor, I was involved in outdoor play projects facilitating wild play sessions with young people. I went on to host wild play sessions for groups, events and gatherings. I would arrive in parks and forests with a toolkit full of string, clay and other creative tools, and we would encourage young people to connect with each other and engage with nature.

Together, we would build intricate clay villages and create forest creatures out of leaves and stones. We would share stories and sip hot chocolate together while taking turns to make wishes with wands made from twigs, feathers and flowers. I was often working with young people who usually struggled to be in a group, and I was in awe of how nature facilitated this compassionate and creative space in which young people could be themselves. I witnessed some incredible and inspiring moments.

When I was 12, I would take myself to the beach to heal and sit on the rocks and look out over the water. I would imagine what it was like to live in the deepest, darkest parts of the ocean and to be able to breathe without drowning. I imagined whole cities under the water, full of sea creatures, kings, queens and protectors. The sea was my calm place, and I would spend hours doodling, drawing and daydreaming as a way to make sense of my own pain and trauma. I remember a particular poem that I wrote called 'Neptune's Kingdom' and it started with these words:

> With my soul worn by the tide, I wander across pearls. I feel the depth of the ocean as she carries my secrets…

This poem went on to explore some of the deepest trauma that I was stuck in and gave real insight into how I was experiencing my life. At the time, I was seeing psychologists and therapists who were struggling to communicate with me, and I have often thought about what a difference it could have made if any one of these professionals had asked me to draw what I was feeling or to write something about what was happening in my inside world.

In nature, how we are feeling on the inside can often be reflected around us on the outside, and if you are thinking about incorporating nature in your counselling practice, I hope that the next few pages will be supportive to you in your work.

> **PRACTICE:** I invite you to take a moment to relax your mind and your body. Maybe you could step outside for a moment and immerse yourself in nature. Now, simply tuning in to your body, I invite you to describe how you are feeling using nature and weather as a metaphor. Describe your 'internal weather' in any way that feels true for you. Maybe you are feeling calm and relaxed like a dreamy, floating cloud, drifting on its path? Or maybe there is something unsettling happening in your life, which feels a bit like a storm approaching. Take a moment to tune in to this and to describe what you are experiencing. If it helps, you could take a moment to draw or write something to explore this further.

CREATIVELY WORKING WITH NATURE AS A CO-THERAPIST

PRACTICE: I invite you to take a moment to connect with nature in the space where you are. Maybe you have a plant in your home or you can walk outside to take in the natural space around you. If you don't have direct access, you could find an image of something from nature online to work with. I invite you to tune in to this image and to connect with the energy in the image. What do you see? What do you feel in your body and where do you feel this? What thoughts are you drawn to? Now imagine that the natural environment has a message for you. What is this message?

When we are working outdoors, we have this incredible environment as a co-therapist. I often like to think of this as Mother Earth working side by side with me to support, nurture and sustain the therapeutic relationship.

In our 'Creative Counsellors Working Creatively in the Outdoors' training module, we explore how the environment becomes the therapy space. We need no tools or resources! We are surrounded by movement, sound, light, energy, texture and imagery to work with. At every turn, a new metaphor presents itself to explore our relationships with ourselves and with the world around us. What an incredible therapy space nature is!

We may come upon an old tree with her leaves falling to the ground, which could open up a conversation around endings and death. We may find ourselves next to a flowing river, offering an opportunity to talk about 'what flow means for the client' or self-care and nurture.

I am excited to share with you some of my favourite ways to work with nature as a co-therapist and I invite you to explore this for yourself before introducing it to clients. You never know what may arise for you.

- *Write a dialogue* – Take a moment to connect with a metaphor from nature that comes to mind and to write a dialogue between you and your metaphor. What message is there for you?
- *Nature doodling* – Find a space in nature to connect with

something that catches your attention. Maybe this is a tree swaying in the wind or maybe it's the tiniest petal of a flower. Take a mindful moment to sketch what you see.

- *Sound bath* – Find a sunny spot in nature and close your eyes to soak up the sounds around you. How does this make you feel?
- *Nature art* – Take some time to collect items in nature on your next outdoor adventure. Find a space to create some nature art and enjoy being in the moment. On reflection, what do you notice about your art? Is there a message for you?
- *Photography* – While out on your walks, take photos of things in nature that catch your attention. What do you see? What stands out for you? A tangled and twisted root. A broken but beautiful old building surrounded by vines. The sun as it rises to nurture our planet.

As you begin to build your practice around working in the outdoors, you will find many new adventures to go on. I hope that, like me, you fall as in love with nature as a therapy space!

> **KEY POINT:** Nature provides us with everything that we need to engage with clients and help them to express their stories, their feelings, their emotions and their experiences.

My Favourite Nature Interventions by Shelby Priestley

Shelby Priestley, a Creative Interventions Therapist, shares her thoughts around working with nature.

I enjoy using nature creatively with clients, both children and adults. Bringing elements of nature into the therapy room can really help clients to find new connections, feel more relaxed and boost their confidence and self-esteem. Being in, or around, nature can improve an individual's mood significantly, which is one of the main reasons I choose to work with nature. I find that clients, both younger and older, have reduced feelings of stress, anxiety and anger after using nature in the therapy room or spending some of our session time outdoors. Working with nature is extremely grounding and can help clients come back to self, as well as experience a state of Mindfulness, which increases their self-awareness.

There are so many ways that you can work with nature in therapy, even if you don't have access to an outdoor area in your practice. Depending on where I am based for each session, I will either ask if clients would like to take our session outside, or I will invite them to use a range of nature resources, such as flowers, leaves, twigs, stones, shells and more during our time together.

I use nature creatively, so will encourage clients to create something using either nature they have collected whilst outside or the nature I have inside the therapy room. The most popular creative activity, I have found, is to use various petals, flowers, leaves, etc. to create a transient piece of art; it can be really powerful. To be able to move and alter their creating freely can be important to clients, as throughout the session, they may feel like something in the picture they have created needs to be moved, adjusted or even taken out. They can also add more to their picture as they go along. At the end of the session, I invite them to take a photo of their art and ask them if they would like to put the picture away or if they would like me to.

This works well with children and young people too, and a firm favourite with younger clients is to use twigs, stones and flowers to create an expression of how they are feeling. This can also be done inside or outside and in the form of transient art.

Another way I use nature in the therapy room is to ask clients to cut a shape of their choice out of cardboard. I use old delivery boxes for this purpose. I then ask them to choose some twine and to wrap the twine around the shape and secure it with some tape or glue.

Again, depending on the location for that session, I will invite clients either to go outside and pick their own flowers or I will have a selection accessible in the room. The activity is to spend some time weaving the flowers through the twine to create a beautiful woven piece of art. I find that this activity usually leads to a comfortable silence, giving the client time to sit with their thoughts and be fully in the moment. This can be a huge positive, and many clients have had a sudden realization about something negative in their life, discovered something about themselves or thought of a solution to a particular obstacle in their life during this activity.

Finally, another popular activity, which while also loved by adults, is enjoyed most by children, is to plant a positive thoughts garden. This activity can get quite messy, so it is best to do it outdoors if you have access. It can be done indoors, but you may need to lay down a mat! Provide the client with some soil, flower seeds and various small decorations, such as glass beads, shells, stones and buttons. Have some paper and pens available too, and a little bit of water. Invite the client to fill up a small tray or flowerpot with soil and to choose a couple of seeds. As they plant the seeds, ask them to think of something positive about themselves. This may be that they are a good friend, they have beautiful eyes or they are a hard worker; anything that feels right to them. When they have watered the seeds, they can begin to decorate the pot or tray as they wish. Tell them that this is their positive thought garden, and by saying out loud one positive thing about themselves every morning, the seeds will grow, and as the flowers grow, so will the client. This is a great way to get them thinking more positively and is a physical reminder, every day, that they are growing as a person – as the amazing individual that they are. The clients are free to take their positive thoughts garden home with them, of course.

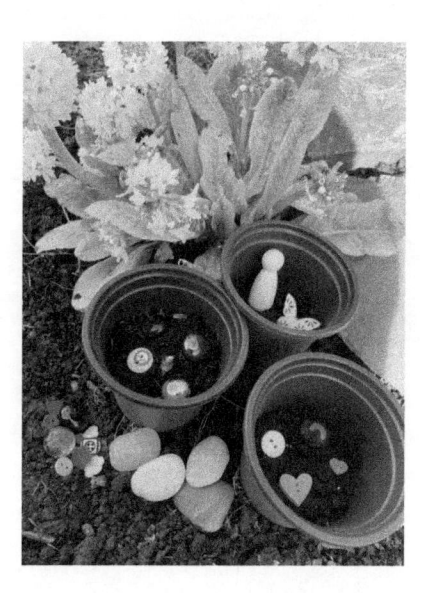

REFLECTIONS

- ❁ Different environments speak to different clients.
- ❁ Some clients find that adjusting the lighting in the room can

have a real impact on their ability to be present, to feel safe and to feel connected.
- Clients will respond differently to different tools and symbols. Having a range of creative tools and symbols that can be used to represent different emotions, life stages, beliefs, interests, genders, values, cultures, life experiences and abilities will help to create a diverse and inclusive space.
- Nature provides us with everything that we need to engage with clients and to help them express their stories, their feelings, their emotions and their experiences.
- Working online can present different challenges for therapists and there may be an increased need for self-care. Don't forget to check in with yourself regularly!

Chapter 3

Relationship and Grounding

Exploring the second element of our Create Circle Approach helps us to think about how we can build and nurture relationships through creative practices, as well as to consider the importance of grounding.

THE FIRST CREATIVE CONNECTION – YOUR MARKETING

I get asked all the time, 'How do I introduce Creative Counselling to my clients?' and I always answer the same way, 'Through your very first interaction together.' This first creative connection may be through your website, a business card, a social media post or a bio on a counsellor directory or database. This may take place via the first email sent or a phone call. However you choose to connect with clients, I invite you to consider how you set the tone for the way that you work from the outset.

Imagine a client not knowing that you work creatively and arriving at your beautiful creative space on day one to find a sea of creative tools and interventions. This could be overwhelming and not what the client expected at all. However, if you share images of your Creative Counselling space and talk transparently about how you work, it is much easier to manage a client's expectations for therapy. I believe that the therapeutic alliance is already starting to be built through this very first connection.

So, How Do We Do This in Practice?

When clients contact me for therapy, one of the first questions I ask is how they came across my details. Many share that they were interested in working with me as my therapist bio is different to others' and that I come across as being more creative and unique in my approach. I am very open about why I work the way that I do and share a little of my own personal story around recovery from sexual violence and other mental health challenges. I have chosen to include details of the way that I work creatively on my website, including exploring my Creative Integrative Approach to therapy and what this means for the client. I believe that the therapeutic alliance is already being formed by my offering transparency, giving a sense of who I am as a therapist and being congruent about what I can and can't offer. I am clear that I am trained in the models of Person-Centred Counselling, Cognitive Behavioural Therapy and Psychodynamic Therapy, and that I have further training in Mindfulness, Neuro-Linguistic Therapy and creative approaches to therapy. This means I take a Holistic and Creative Integrative Approach in which I am unable to single out a specific way of working. So, if a client asks for a purist approach to counselling or is not keen to work creatively, I will always recommend a referral. I feel that this encourages client autonomy and the right to choose what feels good for them in that moment.

With this in mind, your marketing presence is a great way to start to build that creative connection. Think about what images would represent the way that you work. What fonts would share your creative side? What colours represent who you are as a therapist? If you are a creative nature therapist and offer a lot of walk-and-talk counselling, consider images that represent nature and the creative relationship in nature. Maybe a wild garden background or a beautiful tree standing proud, with its roots reaching out with growth.

If you love to work with art, how will your marketing share this with your prospective clients and how do they get a sense of this when they visit your online space? Maybe images of art tables and a nurturing and soothing but creative background and colours. Maybe wild and untamed colours. Anything that represents who you are so that prospective clients can connect with you from the outset.

My branding means that I tend to attract female clients who are drawn to nature and Mindfulness and are looking to explore their situation with a heart-centred, compassionate and gentle approach. I have chosen calming and soothing sand colours, mauves and greens.

PRACTICE: Take a moment to think about who you are as a counsellor. What do you love about what you do and how you work? What are your unique interests and passions in therapy? How can you translate this into your online and marketing presence?

CREATIVE ADDITIONS TO CONTRACTING

Now that your prospective client has found you and experienced that initial connection with you, how do you deepen the creative relationship? The next step in the journey is to consider what additions you can make to your contract to support your clients to understand what creative approaches in counselling you offer and how this might work. In my contract, I have added some additional sections around working creatively and how I offer this. These are reviewed regularly and updated as I shift and adapt the way that I work.

> I am a qualified Integrative Counsellor and Therapeutic Coach, and I am qualified to offer the following therapeutic approaches:
> Creative Approaches in Counselling, Psychodynamic, Person-Centred, CBT, NLP, Hypnotherapy, Mindfulness and Compassion Focused Therapies.
> As a Creative Integrative Counsellor, I draw from all these approaches and offer you an Integrative approach and interventions depending on what you are bringing to each session.

I then go on to explore some of the ways that we could work together.

> Some of the ways that we can work together as a Creative Integrative Counsellor include working with art, clay, poetry, story-making, creative visualizations, Mindfulness, sound, movement, symbols, metaphors, nature walks and any interest and passions that you may have which could support you in your therapy process. During our assessment we can explore these more fully and I would love to answer any questions that you may have.

Now, the client is fully aware of how I work and can make an informed choice about whether they feel that I am the right fit for them; however, I have yet to come across a client who has decided that we are not the right fit at this stage. I believe that this is influenced by how I advertise myself from the outset.

> **KEY POINT:** Your creative connection begins with the very first interaction that your prospective client has with you. This could be your website, your email, your business card or your bio. Explore who you are as a Creative Counsellor and translate this into your marketing presence.

TAKING YOUR CLIENT'S LEAD – 'PACE AND CHECK'

We talk about this often in the counselling world and it is crucially important when working creatively with clients, especially if they are not used to working with creative methods and how impactful and emotive they can be.

Working creatively can take us and our clients down the rabbit hole straight to the unconscious mind within seconds. Our job as therapists is to manage the pace and empower our clients to maintain autonomy within this process. I like to think of this as *pace and check*.

Pacing involves thinking about how our clients are interacting with the creative interventions, and checking involves noticing how this is impacting them. For example, if we begin to notice that our client's anxiety levels are rising and that they appear to be struggling with a sense of feeling overwhelmed, we can support them by actively offering check-in or regrounding moments. We might offer to take a moment to breathe in a safe word or notice three things in the room and describe them. We can discuss openly and own how we are *seeing and sensing* the room.

Example
Counsellor: I have noticed that your shoulders and your fists are tense, you are holding your breath and you seem to be drawn away somewhere. I am wondering what is going on for you right now?

Client: I feel a heaviness in my chest, and I don't like the memories that I am getting right now.

Counsellor: Would it be helpful for us to take a moment to check in and reground ourselves?

Client: Yes please, I just want to shake this off.

Counsellor: So, you are feeling that you want to shake this off. I'm wondering how it would be to literally do as you have intuitively mentioned and shake this off. Shall we do this now?

Client stands and begins to shake arms and body, breathing deeply and moving around the room. Counsellor follows the client's lead, mirroring and reflecting what is being seen. Client sits back down.

Counsellor: How is this for you now?

Client: I feel okay now.

Counsellor: I'm wondering what okay means for you? How is this different than before?

Client: The memories have faded and I don't feel tight in my chest. I feel calm and okay.

Counsellor: What would you like to do now?

Client: I would like to carry on with the exercise.

In this example, the counsellor recognized subtle shifts in the client's body language (checking). Recognizing changes to the rhythm of the breathing, a tightness in the body and some dissociation, the counsellor was able to intuitively support the client to recognize what was happening for them, and by working together, they were able to find their way back into the client's safe zone (pacing). This was helpful in deepening trust and building confidence within the therapeutic relationship.

Deb Dana is one of the leading voices in the therapy field, who talks about the power of Polyvagal Theory. On interviewing her for our Creative Counsellors YouTube channel, I learned about the importance of recognizing shifts in a client's state and how this may be affecting the central nervous system, which could impact on a client's ability to be present and work safely in the session. Deb Dana talks about three states that impact a client in the room.[1]

---

1 www.youtube.com/watch?v=9kv8DdXeoy4

1. When our clients are in a state of 'Ventral Vagal', they feel safe, grounded and socially connected. I interpret this as *I am safe and connected and the world is a safe place.*
2. When clients are in a state of 'Sympathetic or Mobilized', they are in fight or flight mode. I interpret this as *I am in danger and the world is a dangerous place.*
3. When clients are in a state of 'Dorsal Vagal or Immobilized', they are shut down or numb. I interpret this as *I can't cope and the world is too unsafe for me.*

If clients present as feeling emotionally (overwhelmed) or physically (panic attacks) in danger in the therapy session or as if they can't cope (dissociation or numbness), it is our job as therapists to help pace our clients to work within their own window of tolerance – the place and pace that feel safe for them. We can do this by empowering clients with nurturing grounding tools and interventions to support their wellbeing.

> **KEY POINT:** Working creatively can often quickly take clients 'down the rabbit hole' to deeper places. We need to pace and check to make sure that we are facilitating at a pace that meets their needs.

WORKING CREATIVELY WITH GROUNDING TOOLS

Imagine a little boat drifting near a harbour in a calm, turquoise bay. Life feels safe and calm for this little boat. Then, with a flash of lightning and a rumble of thunder, the sea beneath the little boat starts to feel rough. The waters become more turbulent, and the boat begins to feel like it's being tossed and turned in the storm. As the waves begin to crash down around the little boat, it takes a deep breath and knows what it needs to do. It needs to drop anchor. It needs to weather the storm. It knows that it can. It knows that the storm will pass. The little boat drops its anchor and waits out the storm. As the clouds begin to roll away and the seas become calmer, the little boat knows that the storm has passed. The sun begins to peek through the clouds and the little boat begins to feel a sense of calm. The little boat, feeling safe and steady, raises its anchor and begins to drift peacefully again through the harbour.

Just like this little boat, our clients will face their own storms throughout the therapy process. Some storms may feel slightly turbulent, and others could feel overwhelming. It is our job as Creative Counsellors to help our clients prepare for the storm and explore how to drop anchor, creating a solid belief in themselves and that their storm will pass.

Sometimes, the little boat is the client in the room, and at other times, the little boat is the therapist in the room. Having a solid grounding practice is as important for the therapist as it is for the client.

What Is Grounding?

I describe grounding as an anchoring practice that helps to bring a client or us an *in-the-present-moment sense* of physical, emotional and spiritual safety – an in-the-moment awareness and connection to feeling in control.

For many clients who are in therapy, it can be the fear of having a lack of control over emotions or physical sensations in the body during the session that prevents the therapeutic relationship with the therapist and/or self from developing. We can better prepare our clients by guiding them through nurturing grounding practices that support a sense of self-soothing, balance and autonomy.

When we are working creatively in the counselling room, we are often facilitating a multi-sensory approach, which means that there is an innate grounding process that can take place whether we are aware of this or not. We include working with Mind, Body and Feelings by being 'hands on' while exploring the client's story as we invite them to literally 'work through' their experiences. Let's take working with clay as an example. While processing often-complex and sometimes-uncomfortable feelings, the client's hands are grounded in the cooling natural element – moving, expressing and creating. This connection with a natural material, as well as movement and talking, incorporates all the senses – touching the clay, smelling the clay, tasting the subtle hints of earthy flavours in the air, hearing the words that are being shared or the movement of the clay on the surface of the table, seeing the colours as they change shape and are moulded into form, sensing the movement of the body and the space around them. This is all happening at the same time and in the same space.

We are facilitating a deep connection with all the parts of self, and we can witness this unfolding in front of us.

Grounding does, however, mean different things to different people, and we can begin to get a sense of each client's individual Grounding Map when we work creatively to uncover their own interpretation of grounding and what works for them.

Grounding Practice for Clients

Grounding helps clients to feel safe and secure in therapy sessions. This is especially helpful for clients who dissociate in the room or struggle to be present. For those clients who struggle with anxiety, flashbacks and panic attacks, having an understanding of how to work with the central nervous system to gain a sense of control can feel very empowering.

Carrying out a grounding assessment early in the therapeutic relationship can be a useful way to begin to create a safe space for therapy.

PRACTICE: Your Grounding Map: I invite you to take a moment right now to get comfortable. So comfortable that you notice how nice it feels to be sitting or lying where you are. Closing your eyes, I invite you to think of someone or somewhere that brings you a sense of safety. Staying with this for a moment, notice what you notice. How do you know that you feel safe? Can you describe this? How does this feel in your body? What emotions represent feeling safe for you?

Take a moment to write, doodle or draw this out for you.

You have begun to create your own Grounding Map.

EXAMPLE

Therapist: Take a moment to get really comfortable. So comfortable that you notice how nice this feels. Let me know when you are relaxed and comfortable.

Client: Okay.

Therapist: Closing your eyes, I now invite you to think of someone or somewhere that brings you a feeling of safety.
Client: I have it.
Therapist: Is this someone or somewhere?
Client: Somewhere and someone. My bed and my teddy.
Therapist: Your bed and your teddy. How do you know that you feel really safe in your bed with your teddy? Do you feel this in your body?
Client: Because I feel calm and relaxed.

Helping our clients to tune in to what feeling safe means to them helps to create a vision, a feeling and a sense of safety that they can draw on if needed in the future. It's important to note that it is best to facilitate this while the client is in a place of safety, calm and connection. It is much more difficult to explore what helps a client to feel grounded when they are in the middle of the storm, experiencing overwhelm, dissociation, triggers or flashbacks.

Some clients may describe things in detail and others may use one or two words.

Grounding Words

We now know that the client in the example above can relate to grounding using the words 'feeling calm and relaxed'. Grounding words are a useful tool for guiding clients to connect with that sense of safety when needed. You can gently remind clients of their words as a statement. You can help clients to connect with those feelings and to return to a place of feeling anchored and in control.

Grounding words can be anything, anywhere or anyone. Some clients may choose words that represent their loved ones, tuning in to that feeling of being held safely in the arms of another. Other clients may choose words that describe a colour that reminds them of a place, like a forest or their childhood home. Some clients may choose to work with images and describe words based on what they are seeing. I have experienced clients bringing an image of their pets into the therapy room and we have created describing words around these images.

EXAMPLE

Client: Benji helps me to feel safe. He's my dog. I have a picture on my phone. Can I show you?

Therapist: Benji sounds important to you. I would like to see him.

Client: He isn't actually with us any more as he died two years ago. But I know that he is really with me all the time in spirit. I know he protects me and I can still sometimes smell him in the room after I take a walk.

Therapist: So, you have a real sense of him being with you and protecting you. You can smell him around you after you take a walk. Can you describe how having Benji with you like this helps to create that sense of safety?

Client: He was always very protective of me. He loved me no matter what I did. Even when I wasn't being fair. He never judged me. He is what real unconditional love is.

Therapist: So, feeling real unconditional love from Benji. Feeling that he is protective and he is there for you. Can you feel this anywhere in your body while we are talking? Can you tune in to this feeling for a moment?

Client: Yes. I feel it in my throat, in my stomach and in the top of my head.

Therapist: And what does this feel like?

Client: It feels warm and like it's swirling.

Grounding Visualizations

Grounding visualizations can help us to support clients to be very present in the here and now, and they are particularly useful when clients are struggling with the symptoms of PTSD, dissociation, anxiety and generalized anxiety. Working with the whole body and the brain, we can invite clients to literally visualize their safe place – being rooted strong and steady like a tree or drifting gently along on a cloud. These practices help to distract clients from other thoughts and feelings, as well as supporting them to be 'in the room'.

EXAMPLE

Therapist: I invite you to place both feet on the floor and find your most comfortable seated position. Take a moment to sink into your chair until you are ready, then let me know.

Client: Okay, I'm feeling comfortable.

Therapist: Maybe closing your eyes if that feels okay for you and imagining a beautiful, strong and steady tree standing in the middle of a lush and green field. Can you see this?

Client: Yes, it's tall and the sun is coming through the leaves.

Therapist: As the sun shines down through the leaves, can you feel that warmth too?

Client: I can. It feels nice.

Therapist: What else do you notice about this tree?

Client: It's tall and strong.

Therapist: I want to invite you to imagine now that you are the tree. Tall and strong. Steady and rooted. Your feet are connected to the earth. Your body is balanced and safe. Your branches are filled with sunlight. How does that feel?

Client: I feel relaxed and strong. I feel like my roots are really deep.

Therapist: Notice how deep your roots are and how strong you are, just like this tree. Taking some deep, relaxing breaths, and when you are ready, open your eyes.

We can see from this example that this client is very visual and responds well to these kinds of prompts. At this point, the therapist could invite the client to draw the tree or create a grounding statement together to deepen the experience even more. There is always a natural next step to work with when we are taking the client's lead.

Breathing and Focusing on the Breath

Focusing on how our breath feels as it is entering and leaving the body can help to strengthen the grounding process. We can invite clients simply to notice how the breath enters through the mouth and the nose and the route it takes all the way to the stomach. To notice what it feels like to shift the breath to a more relaxed count or expand the stomach as it fills with air. One of my favourite ways to support clients to focus on their breathing is to invite them to breathe in naturally in a way that feels good to them while taking their time to breathe out as if they are blowing bubbles. Clients may naturally begin to focus on the outbreath, and as this happens, we can begin to draw their attention to creating a longer outbreath. Over the years, I have begun to notice the subtle changes in how a client's body posture softens as they start to take longer outbreaths. Their face muscles relax, their shoulders drop down and they begin to melt into the moment. This is a great intervention to facilitate as we are building a client's toolbox of new skills that they can turn to in any moment of need.

Colour Bubble Breathing

I remember lying in bed as a child and being too scared to sleep. I would lie awake for hours and stare at the shadows in the room or listen for noises outside my windows. We were living in South Africa, and it was a particularly turbulent and worrying time, with many break-ins and violent crimes taking place around us. We would often hear guard dogs barking in the distance; sometimes gunfire would explode like fireworks and I would tune in to every tiny sound and wait for something bad to happen to our family. I lived in a near - constant state of alert.

While navigating these traumatic times, I was drawn to art and colour. I would create vibrant drawings and decorate my room with colour to create what I now recognize as a safe sanctuary away from the fear outside.

My mom would tuck me in and ask me to think of a colour that felt safe and loving. I would choose pinks or greens or blues. She would invite me to breathe in these colours and to surround myself in bubbles of colour. I would relax totally into her arms and into my warm duvet. I remember waking often in the night and imagining myself surrounded in my safe bubble of sea-green light. Sea green was my favourite colour because I always felt safe at the beach. I loved to watch the ocean.

EXAMPLE

Let's explore how to facilitate Colour Bubble Breathing with clients.

Therapist: Take a moment to think of a colour that feels safe and loving to you.

Client: Okay, definitely pink.

Therapist: Is it any specific shade of pink or pink as a whole.

Client: I love a really vibrant hot pink.

Therapist: So, a really vibrant hot pink.

Client: Yes!

Therapist: I invite you to close your eyes for a moment and to begin to imagine a bubble of vibrant hot-pink energy starting to surround you. Can you see or feel this?

Client: Yes, it started at my feet and is moving upwards.

Therapist: Allow this colour to continue to move upwards until it surrounds your whole body. Notice how it feels to be in this safe and loving energy.

Client: It feels warm and relaxing.

Therapist: So, warm and relaxing.

Client: Yes.

Therapist: Now notice that with each breath you take, how you are breathing this colour bubble into your body, too. A bubble of vibrant hot-pink, warm and relaxing energy. Notice what you notice.

Client: It feels soothing and clearing.

Therapist: When you are ready, begin to notice how your pink bubble begins to move back down around you and to your feet. Knowing that you can come back to this bubble any time that you want.

You may have noticed how, in this example, the therapist adapts their exercise to incorporate the words and phrases that the client uses. This helps the client to take ownership of their process and will support them in a nurturing and safe way.

Sand-Tray Grounding

If you are working with sand in the therapy room, a beautiful way to offer grounding in the sand is to invite the client to create shapes and patterns in the sand using their fingers, hands and objects.

Invite clients simply to focus on the feeling of the sand between their fingers as it falls back into the tray or create intricate patterns and movement. Sand can feel very nurturing for clients, often tapping into that inner child 'Peter Pan' part of us that waits to be invited to play.

This soothing practice draws on visual, kinaesthetic and auditory elements, which offers a full body and holistic experience for the client.

When we engage with all the senses, we can really help our clients to be grounded and in the present moment.

MIND, BODY, FEELINGS AND INTUITION (MBFI)

Mind - Body - Feelings - Intuition

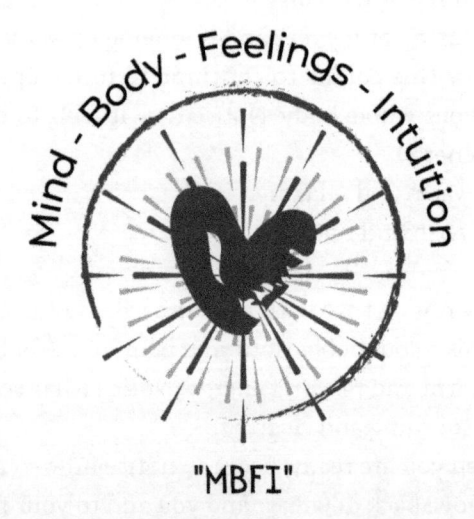

"MBFI"

I created this Mind, Body, Feelings and Intuition (MBFI) Cycle in 2018 as we started to facilitate trainings around creativity in counselling. In my work as a trauma counsellor, I became aware of how important it is to work with the whole person and the whole experience – to include the body and any spiritual and intuitive awareness, as well as the mind and the feelings. This is incredibly powerful as a noticing, mirroring and reflecting exercise to help clients to bring awareness to their own way of being, processes and therapeutic shifts.

- *Mind* – What is happening with our clients' thoughts, thinking patterns and beliefs, and what impact this is having on the creative process.
- *Body* – What the client is actually experiencing physically in the body. Any shifts and changes, and bringing awareness to this.
- *Feelings* – What emotions and feelings a client is aware of and how this is impacting on or informing the exercise.
- *Intuition* – Any spiritual, intuitive or other energy shifts that

may be taking place, and actively supporting the client to explore these.

Example

Counsellor: I'm wondering whether there is a word that describes that image for you?

Client: I *think* [mind] it's broken.

Counsellor: Broken. I noticed that you sat back as you said that. I'm wondering what you may be sensing or feeling physically in your body?

Client: I'm *feeling a cold swirling in my stomach* [body], round about here.

Counsellor: So, you are feeling a cold, swirling in your stomach round about here. I'm wondering if there is an emotion to describe what this feels like?

Client: Um, sadness [feeling]. Deep, deep sadness.

Counsellor: Deep, deep sadness. *Takes a deep breath*. I'm wondering what we could say to that sadness that it needs to hear, if anything?

Client: It's okay. You are not alone. I am here for you. You are not alone. *Points up to the sky*.

Counsellor: It's okay, you are not alone. I am here for you. You are not alone. And I noticed that you pointed up to the sky.

Client: I believe that God [intuition] wants me to know that I am not alone.

Counsellor: God wants you to know that you are not alone. And how is this different for you now?

Client: I feel calm and safe. I know that I am okay.

As we can see in this example, the counsellor guided the client creatively through all four elements of the MBFI Cycle. Mirroring, noticing, reflecting, checking and pacing.

CHECK IN, CREATIVE PROCESS, CHECK OUT

CHECK IN – CREATIVE PROCESS – CHECK OUT

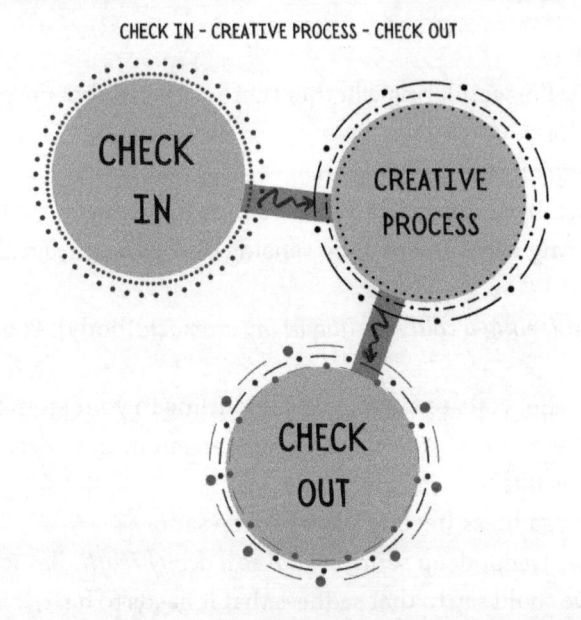

We have spoken about just how powerful working creatively can be, and I have found that a three-step framework helps me to support the client throughout the process. No matter how I am working with the client, I tend to work within the same frame.

1. *Check in* – Usually around 5–10 minutes. At the beginning of each session, I check in with the client to clarify what they would like from the session. I offer some grounding interventions and reminders, and we explore where the client would like to start.
2. *Creative process* – Usually around 35–40 minutes. During this stage, we explore whatever the client brings in the way that they would like to work. Talking, playing, art, creating, moving or any other creative intervention that therapeutically supports the client and meets their needs.
3. *Check out* – Usually around 5–10 minutes. During this stage, I will literally 'check out' where the client is, offering grounding interventions where necessary and reconnecting with the here and now. What does my client need to leave the room

emotionally and physically safe today? Are there any safeguarding concerns to take action on? Is there anything else that I need to consider here?

KNOWING WHEN TO PIVOT OR SHIFT EXERCISE

There may be times when you are facilitating a creative exercise and you begin to notice or sense an energy shift in the client, a change in the relationship with the intervention or something that catches your attention. I have learned that it's important to say what I see in these circumstances and to own what I am sensing – going back to checking and pacing.

Sometimes, you may have identified a creative intervention together that could support the client to express or explore something that is important for them. You may have offered this to other clients before and you may think, 'Well, this usually takes around 20 minutes to complete', but for some reason today your client is 5 minutes into the exercise and something just isn't feeling like it's in flow. That sense of something being a little 'off' for your client – I would invite you to address this and to own your feelings so that your client has the opportunity to check in with themselves too. The ebb and flow is part of the process, and you will have days when things seem to flow and other days when the interaction is a little more prickly to manage. Engaging with your client to share what you are noticing often empowers them to be autonomous and to take control of their own process. I often find that when my 'spidey senses' are intuitively tingling deep down in my belly, this is a call to act. A simple statement like, 'I am sensing that something has changed for you – how are you finding this exercise at the moment?' or even, 'I noticed that you have moved away from the clay and I'm wondering what's happening for you now?'. There are a number of reasons why you may be sensing a change in the room; here are some examples.

- ✪ The client can't relate to the exercise and may need some support.
- ✪ They may be nervous and fearful of not being creative enough or of judgement.

- They may have already had some conscious awareness of what they need to work with, and this exercise may not suit this shift in awareness.
- They may be experiencing a traumatic trigger of some kind.
- They may feel too tired to continue or need the toilet and not want to say so.
- They may not want to be creative today.
- Something else may have come up that they want to explore.

Checking in and providing space for exploration in the room often helps to nurture the relationship and build confidence in the client's trust in the creative process. It's also an important ethical consideration and helps to keep the work within the client's frame of reference, ultimately meeting their needs, facilitating their goals and empowering them to lead.

> **KEY POINT:** Say what you see and share what you are feeling. Don't be afraid to explore, shift and pivot between exercises if need be. Take a Peter Pan approach to being playful and curious.

Grounding Practice for Counsellors

When we talk about grounding tools, it's easy to forget that counsellors need to have a solid grounding practice just as much as clients. For us to be the steady and stable lighthouse in the room, guiding clients safely back to shore, we need to recognize how to practise self-care in a way that replenishes our own stores of energy and promotes healing and wellbeing for ourselves.

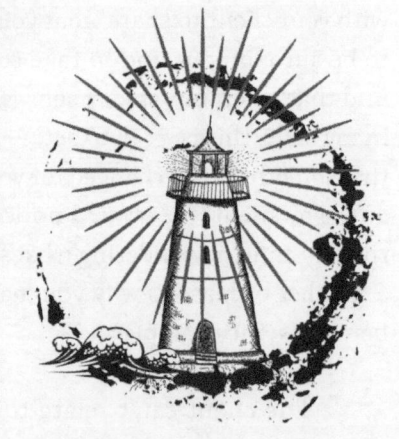

Grounding helps us as counsellors to restore and re-energize our systems. It can help us to take time to reflect on the day and our work. Being in a grounded place helps us to bounce back from challenging situations and provides us with the opportunity to find balance in our personal and professional lives. Without a self-care and/or grounding practice, we can easily find ourselves in a place of burnout or vicarious trauma.

In 2017, I experienced first-hand how harmful it was not to have a grounding practice, and I paid a heavy price for this. At the time, I was balancing both a full caseload of clients in my role as a counsellor working for a specialist trauma service and a busy private practice. The work that I was doing was specialized, and I began to develop a reputation for being able to support a niche set of clients who at the time did not have many services to count on. As a result, I was operating with a long waiting list, I had daily emails to filter through, and I struggled to find any balance and maintain boundaries. I would wake up in the mornings feeling as tired as I did when I went to bed, and my life felt like it was always speeding up. I started to struggle to find time to be social with family and friends and always prioritized work. When I was spending any time being social, I struggled to connect with people who weren't in trauma. I was totally disconnected from talking about everyday things like movies or holidays. My mind would always wander back to my therapy room. I was surrounding myself with therapy books, and my idea of self-care was to take a bath while listening to a therapy podcast. I watched movies about hard-hitting topics related to my work and answered emails during dinner time. My family started to voice their concerns, and I thought that I was just a hard worker. What I didn't know was that I was beginning to slide down the slippery slope into burnout. My lantern light was slowing dimming. My reserves of energy were being depleted, and I began to feel unplugged! I wasn't able to recharge, and all my systems were misfiring. As I became more and more exhausted, I started to struggle with unexplained pains, mind fog, extreme tiredness, inability to digest foods properly, itching and sensitive skin, blurry eyes and heaviness in my body. I felt like my arms had become heavy weights and they couldn't carry any more. I felt as though my ears could not hear any more, and every day I struggled with sore throats. My body was telling me and showing me that I had no grounding, nurturing or self-care practice. Or that whatever practice I currently had wasn't working for me.

Recovering from this deep burnout was going to take time. I had to begin again to explore what raised me up. What filled my cup. What gave me a sense of balance and helped me to be energized and in a place of calm confidence. It took years to be able to connect the dots fully, but I came to find that I could create my own personal grounding routine or map to bring more balance into my world.

- *Supportive people* – Spending time with people who challenge me from a place of love, nurture me and celebrate my wins with me. Those who are non-judgemental and give as much as they take. I surround myself with incredible people who are having a positive impact on the world, and this feels good.
- *Places in nature* – Finding space and time to be in nature. Exploring my adventurous side. Travelling and connecting with new places. Swimming in rivers, walking in beautiful spaces, sitting in silence in the sun, growing beautiful plants and feeling a deep sense of connection to my place in our ecosystem. I see myself as a tree that needs nurturing, a place to root and a space to grow.
- *Daily spiritual practice* – Taking time daily to explore my spiritual side, including meditation, practising gratitude, breathing and relaxation exercises. More time to focus on my purpose and my passions in life.
- *Time to be creative* – I found that the more I found space to be creative for no reason, the more energy I started to regain. I now have doodle books, scrapbooks and a dedicated creativity space at home in the garden. I can tune in to this whenever I feel the need for some self-expression.
- *Taking off my professional hat* – The hardest job I had was to retrain my brain to take off my professional hat everyday so that I could return to being a mother, a partner and a person before a professional, but this took time. A few years ago, during a particularly challenging time in my counselling work, I noticed that I was struggling to maintain boundaries between my personal and professional life. I was answering emails late into the night and accepting new bookings for appointments on weekends even though I had agreed with my family that I

wouldn't, and it was becoming more and more difficult to be fully present during family time. My partner called me out on this, which led me to working with a therapist who specializes in work stress. During this time, I recognized that I was feeling a sense of needing to 'do more' to help all the clients who were finding their way to my inbox daily. I had to make some changes or I was going to burn out quickly, which was going to affect my health and my relationships. So, I decided to limit my appointments in the day to four, to take Fridays off so I had a three-day weekend and to use a separate phone for work-related enquiries. These small changes helped to create some separation in my roles, which has had a positive and uplifting effect on all aspects of my life. It starts with reflecting on what your needs are and what drives you, and then reaching out for support if you need this!

- *Practising self-compassion* – One of the biggest gifts I have ever given myself is the gift of self-compassion. Treating myself in the way that I would treat a good friend or a tiny little puppy that needs nurturing. Allowing myself the space to explore; to make mistakes and to be free to make new choices. Being okay with saying no and knowing that I matter too. My health and wellbeing is just as important as the health and wellbeing of my clients. Forgiving myself for any moments when I may forget this.

What I mostly learned was how to tune in to my own inner compass, to trust my instincts, and to learn to work with my intuition and felt sense in the body. This has enabled me to begin to find a renewed sense of what grounding is for me personally.

> **KEY POINT:** As Creative Counsellors, we can utilize the same creative approach that we offer our clients to tune in to ourselves and hear the messages that the body wants to share with us to create our own Grounding Map.

Your unique Grounding Map or blueprint might also include rituals and routines for when you are working with clients in the room. Some of my favourite ground practices include:

- washing my hands and taking a drink of water in between clients
- writing my thoughts out if I need to process anything that affected me or came up during a session
- walking outside after a tricky session or listening to some music
- jumping up and down on the spot and literally 'shaking off' any unpleasant sensations
- opening windows to let fresh air in to re-energize my mind, ready for my next client
- taking more time between clients and pacing my sessions out over the week to make sure that I have time to pursue other passions in life
- referring clients on when I need to and taking regular holidays and breaks.

PRACTICE: Take a moment to connect with the people, places and things that ground you in life. What and who helps you to feel nurtured, safe and restored?

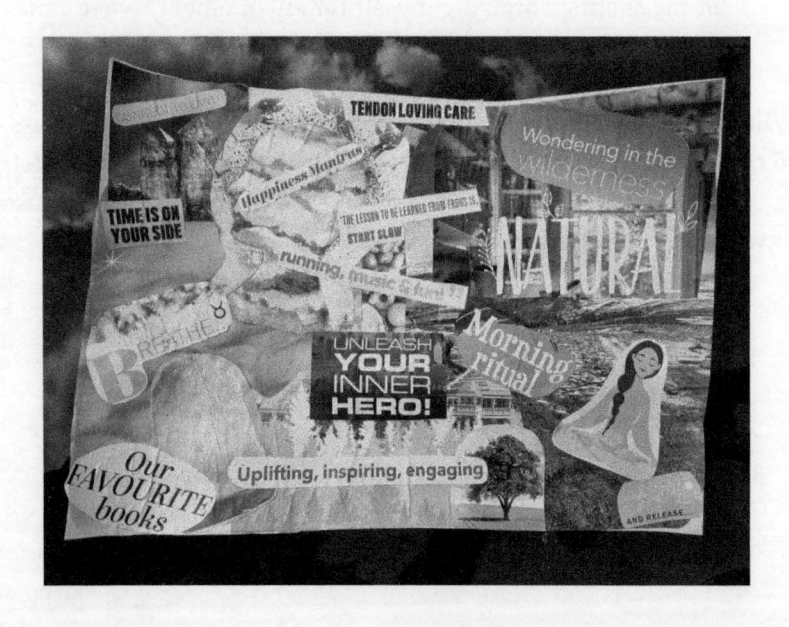

REFLECTIONS

- Your creative connection begins with the very first interaction that your prospective client has with you. This could be your website, your email, your business card or your bio. Explore who you are as a Creative Counsellor and translate this into your marketing presence.
- Working creatively can often take clients 'down the rabbit hole' to deeper places quickly. We need to pace and check to make sure that we are facilitating at a pace that meets their needs.
- Say what you see and share what you are feeling. Don't be afraid to explore, shift and pivot between exercises if need be. Take a Peter Pan approach to being playful and curious.
- Remember the MBFI model and to reflect on Mind, Body, Feelings and Intuition throughout the process.
- Take some time to check in, create and check out with the client.

Chapter 4

Engage and Evaluate

CREATIVE INTERVENTIONS TO HELP ENGAGE THE CLIENT IN THE GOALS-SETTING PROCESS

In this chapter, we will explore different creative examples of how we can engage with the client to evaluate their goals and work with their interests within the Creative Counselling process. We will also explore how to work safely to support clients who may have experienced past trauma.

CREATIVE ASSESSMENTS

PRACTICE: Take a moment to think about an area of your life that you would like to change or improve. Maybe this is related to work, relationships, health or something else. Start to explore this by drawing, doodling, writing or creating something that represents where you are now and where you would like to get to. Once you have created this, think about what could help you to build a bridge between where you are now and where you would like to be. Reflect on this and consider how you can action this in your life.

I used to work with form-based and tick-box-style assessment tools until I realized that my clients would often tell me what they thought I needed to hear in these assessments. Clients would often share that they felt they had to add 'numbers' to their forms to appear more anxious or depressed than they actually were, as they had been waiting for help for so long and were fearful of being pushed to the back of the list.

I also found that as we moved through the therapy process, clients would sometimes become stuck on the numbers and would identify how they were improving by their scores instead of how their life was being impacted. I had clients who would overestimate positive numbers, as they wanted to leave on a 'high' and didn't want to offend me.

I was left with a feeling of unease about working with forms, and we now know that many counsellors are stepping away from forms and looking for more creative ways to assess clients throughout the work.

We can also use creative engagement and assessment interventions to understand more about why clients have come to therapy, what their goals are and who the silent stakeholders are in the room, such as loved ones or significant important people.

> **KEY POINT:** Many clients benefit from assessments that don't involve 'ticking the box' or 'scoring points'. Creative assessments help us to explore the client's needs and desired outcomes for therapy through a more natural and relaxed approach.

MY LIFE CIRCLE

In this exercise, I invite clients to draw a circle (or any shape) on their sheet of paper as a starting point. Then, we work together to explore how we can break this up into smaller chunks that represent different areas of struggle that a client would like to work on in therapy. This might include people, relationships, work, career, finances, creativity, spontaneity, health and wellbeing, or anything that the client feels is important.

Once we have created the outline, I invite the client to give each section a number, word or symbol that represents how significantly this issue is impacting on their life. By doing this, we begin to identify the most important areas to focus on, and we can begin to explore where the client would like to start in the therapy work.

This also works well as a My Feelings Circle or even a My Limiting-Beliefs Circle where the focus might be on the thoughts and beliefs that the client holds about their life and self that are most affecting them right now.

WORKING WITH NUMBER-RANGE ASSESSMENTS

The assessment below is a simple verbal check-in that help us to explore an 'in-the-moment' feeling, presenting issue, goal or emotion. It works with a range of numbers from 0 to 10.

Example

Counsellor: I hear you say that you have carried this anxiety with you for most of your life. I am wondering on a scale of 0–10, where 0 is nothing at all and 10 is enormous, what sort of impact has this had on your life so far?

Client: 8.

Counsellor: 8 can mean different things for different people and I'm wondering what this number means for you?

Client: It means that I can't really go outside or do anything as I am scared of being judged because I have autism.

Counsellor: So, you feel as though you can't really go outside or do anything as you are feeling scared of being judged and this feels like an 8?

Client: Yes!

Counsellor: I'm wondering if this ever gets to a 10?

Client: Yes, one time someone at school laughed at me and took a video of me tripping over and shared this with the whole school with #autistic. That was the worst day and it felt like a 10.

Counsellor: I am wondering. as we have 12 weeks to work together, what number might represent feeling like you could maybe go outside and do something without feeling scared of being judged?

Client: I think maybe a 4. That would feel okay. I don't want to say a 3 as it feels too hard and I don't want any pressure.

Counsellor: Thank you for sharing this with me. So, a 4 feels like it might be achievable. Just playing with numbers here, what happens if it's like a 5 or a 3? What would that mean for you at the end of therapy?

Client: That would be okay.

So, in this example, the counsellor is checking where the client is at through numbers, giving the client their own frame of reference for how they are feeling and where they would like to get to in therapy. It's also helped to identify some goals and a starting point. The counsellor checked how flexible the client is around numbers, as it is important not to get too tied up around the outcome or to be too fixed on the numbers. If this were to happen, an important conversation around numbers would be encouraged to create some more understanding of the process of counselling.

> **KEY POINT:** Working with numbers is a quick and easy way to reflect on where the client is in the moment. This can help to identify triggers, changes and transitions in the client's state and to evaluate the process.

SAND-TRAY FAMILIES AND RELATIONSHIPS

When evaluating where a client may be in their circle, symbols can be a powerful ally. You can invite the client to explore your symbols and select any that represent people that come to mind who are involved in their world. These can be people from the past or the present; I have even had future people appear in the tray when exploring relationships, love and friendships.

You can explore the qualities of these people and how they impact on the client. Think about the placement of the symbols and the size of the symbols.

What could a large angry-looking gorilla standing directly behind the small butterfly mean for the client? Who does the client's symbol have in their line of sight and who do they not see in the tray?

You can invite the client to introduce their tray to you and to walk you through their symbols. Use a gentle inquiry approach such as, 'I'm wondering which symbol you are most drawn to in the tray right now and why?'. Who isn't in the tray and why?

It's incredible how quickly we can get to know a client's world by working in this way compared with a talking approach.

A HOPES-AND-DREAMS BOARD

This is a particularly popular exercise with teen clients, as they are empowered to explore their hopes and dreams through photos, images, colour and words. I always keep a good stash of magazines with me so I can work with collage, as it's a sticky, playful and light touch to start with.

Invite your client to create a collage that represents their hopes and dreams; this can be done on paper or card, in a journal or digitally on a laptop, tablet or computer. It's such a versatile assessment and evaluation tool.

Invite your client to select how they would like to create their collage; offering a few suggestions may help. They can collect, cut, shred and organize a selection of images that they are drawn to working with. Invite your client to add any words, colours, phrases, elements or anything else that they would like to.

Explore this with your client to make sense of their goals and dreams.

Example

Counsellor: I'm wondering if you could talk me through your hopes-and-dreams board.

Client: I like blue and so there's a lot of blues on there. Most people feel blue when they are down, but I feel blue when I am feeling calm and relaxed. I also have some people on there as I haven't seen my friends for a while because I don't go to school at the moment because of my depression. I have some sunshine because I know that if I can start to go to school again and see my friends then I will feel brighter. I have added some shells because I want to study to work with marine animals and I know that if I can sort out my depression then I will be able to do this, and also I have to first finish school, which is a big challenge for me. I wanted to put a red heart on my page but I don't like the colour red because it reminds me of blood and I don't want to think about that.

Counsellor: Thank you for sharing that with me. I'm hearing that school is a big challenge for you right now and I'm getting a sense that you feel that if you can get back to school then this will help you and that red is definitely a colour that you don't like?

Client: Yes, and I miss it.

Within one exercise, the counsellor already knows a lot about this young person, including their goals, some fears and also some hopes for the future. The counsellor will often also have been unconsciously and consciously receiving a lot more information from the client, for example how long they take to explore and process information, anything that the client reacted to in the magazines, specific body language phrases and other interests that may pop up. There was also a trigger colour there that I would add to my notes if a client shared this in the session.

EVALUATING TRIGGERS

When we are working creatively, it is important to note any triggers that a client has that could be traumatizing for them. I have been in the room when a counsellor has offered an intervention to a client around masks and found out a few minutes in that their client is terrified of masks. In my experience, clients won't often share their triggers with us unless we ask them to; often this is because of a sense of being judged or having experiences in the past in which their feelings and fears haven't been validated. With this in mind, I am always upfront with this question when it feels right and we are getting to know each other. As I work in a trauma-informed way, I will often include this with some psychoeducation around trauma and trauma triggers.

Example

'When we work creatively, it can help for me to know if there are any things that might trigger your anxiety or make you feel uncomfortable. For example, if you have a fear of ice cream, then I wouldn't want to create a visualization for you based around ice cream as that wouldn't feel very relaxing. I'm wondering if there are any colours, outdoor places, animals, feelings, trigger words or anything that I should be aware of so I can support you?'

DOODLING, SKETCHING AND DRAWING

One of the simplest and most effective creative assessment approaches is to invite clients to explore with a pen and paper to share their thoughts and feelings through words, colours, shapes, patterns and lines.

Example

- 'I'm wondering if you could doodle something on that sheet of paper to express how you are feeling right now in this moment?'
- 'You mention that you want to feel more confident, I'm wondering whether you could doodle what this means for you? How will you know that you feel more confident?'
- 'You shared that you wanted to show me how important this is to you but you don't know how to tell me, and I'm wondering whether you could draw this instead using shapes, symbols, patterns, colours and lines?'

NATURE METAPHORS

Incorporating nature metaphors into our assessment process can help some clients to express themselves through images, sounds and elements found in nature.

Example

- 'I'm feeling as angry as lightning.'
- 'My anxiety sounds as loud as a woodpecker in my head.'
- 'I am as prickly as a cactus.'
- 'She was as trustworthy as a snake.'
- 'I am as nervous as a caged lion.'
- 'Life feels as hopeless as a choking tree.'

This can also provide clients with some distance, which might help them to talk and remain within their safe zone or their window of tolerance.

FROM-HERE-TO-THERE EXERCISE

This is my personal favourite tool and I always gain so much insight from it. I invite the client to divide their paper in half in any way that they like. Once it's divided, I invite the client to represent themselves and their current life on one side. Then I invite the client to represent how they would like to see themselves and experience life on the other side of the sheet.

The real magic is in drawing the bridge between them and inviting the client to explore all the things they think could help them to 'bridge the gap'.

I've found this to be a very powerful exercise for clients!

TOOLS TIMELINE

I introduce the concept of the Tools Timeline to new clients towards the end of the first session. I ask them to choose a symbol, word, sentence, colour or anything that represents that session and record this on a sheet of paper. They may want to add interventions that helped or something that will nudge their memory in the future. We do this at the end of each session, and by the final session, we have a full timeline as a reminder of the client's therapeutic process. Some clients like to take this away with them and others like to leave it with their notes.

For example, in session 3, your client may have explored setting boundaries and uncovered that saying 'no' was not as scary as they first thought. This could be a great addition to their Tools Timeline:

Session 3: 'I can assert my boundaries and saying no is important.'

Or in session 5, they may have learned a new breathing technique that empowers them to relax their body when experiencing a flashback:

Session 5: 'I can breathe through and take control of my flashbacks! 1, 2, 3, 4, 5, 6, 7, 8, 9, 10.'

Then, in the last session, we have a timeline as a reminder of the therapeutic process for the clients. Some clients like to take this away with them and others like to leave them with their notes.

This is a great way to assess the client throughout the sessions, especially if they are adding numbers or emotion words as they move through their weeks with you. By supporting clients to add all these elements to their Tools Timeline session by session, you are empowering them to access these skills confidently if they need them in the future.

Celebrating your journey

www.creativecounsellors.org

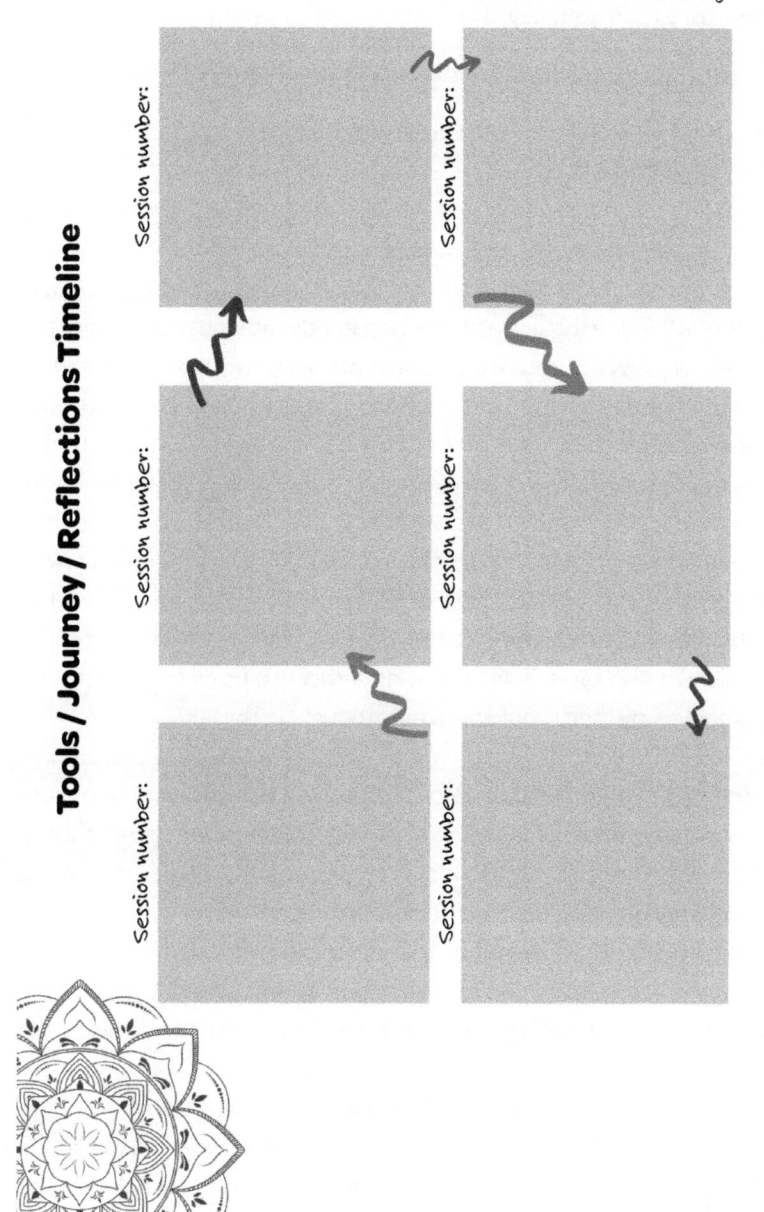

Tools / Journey / Reflections Timeline

Session number:
Session number:
Session number:
Session number:
Session number:
Session number:

This worksheet is available to download from https://library.jkp.com/redeem using the voucher code: VLAJAFS

> **KEY POINT:** Keeping a record of the client's journey, including any shifts, creative skills and tools that they have acquired along the way, can be a powerful part of the process for clients to recognize their journey.

My World Creative Assessment Tool by Kemi Omijeh

Kemi Omijeh, a Creative Child and Adolescent Therapist, shares her 'My World Creative Assessment tool' with us.

I have a range of creative tools that I use to engage children; this particular tool is the one that I use most consistently with most of my clients. I describe it as a way to capture a snapshot of their world. It is quite a simple idea that can be built on in so many different ways. It comes alive and looks different with each child's interpretation of it. This is one of the things I enjoy about working creatively with children and young people: I plant the seed, they run with it. The resource has changes with each client, because they all give me ideas. So, for example, I had a client humming a tune as we were working on their world, which gave me the idea of adding the question: What would be the soundtrack playing to accompany your world? Another client made their world 3D and moveable using card and pipe cleaners – a much more creative way than I could have ever thought of myself.

I present the client with a template of five circles. The core circle represents them; I tell them they can draw themselves, bring a favourite picture of themselves or simply fill it with their favourite colour. Some clients choose simply to write their name. I also include pronouns, as it's important to be inclusive in my practice, but also because it presents an opportunity for a client to tell me how they identify in the first session without me making any assumptions. The other circles represent home, family, friends, and school and college. The template is a visual that helps me explain the activity; I then ask them how they would like to create theirs. They can fill in the template or we can create one from scratch in whatever way they would like.

There are question prompts for each circle, but I always tell the young person that these are just guidance and they can include or exclude what they like. Depending on how much I know about the client, I adjust the question prompts to what is suitable. The question prompts I choose inform my ongoing assessment and give a creative way to explore a client's identity and their personal life and background. The questions about their world help me to join the dots of their life; often the clients are joining the dots, too. There's something about seeing your world/representations of your world concretely in front of you. If the timing is right and it feels appropriate, I also use it as a descriptive metaphor for what therapy can be about – not just to address challenges and difficulties but also to join the dots and allow them a safe space to explore different parts of themselves.

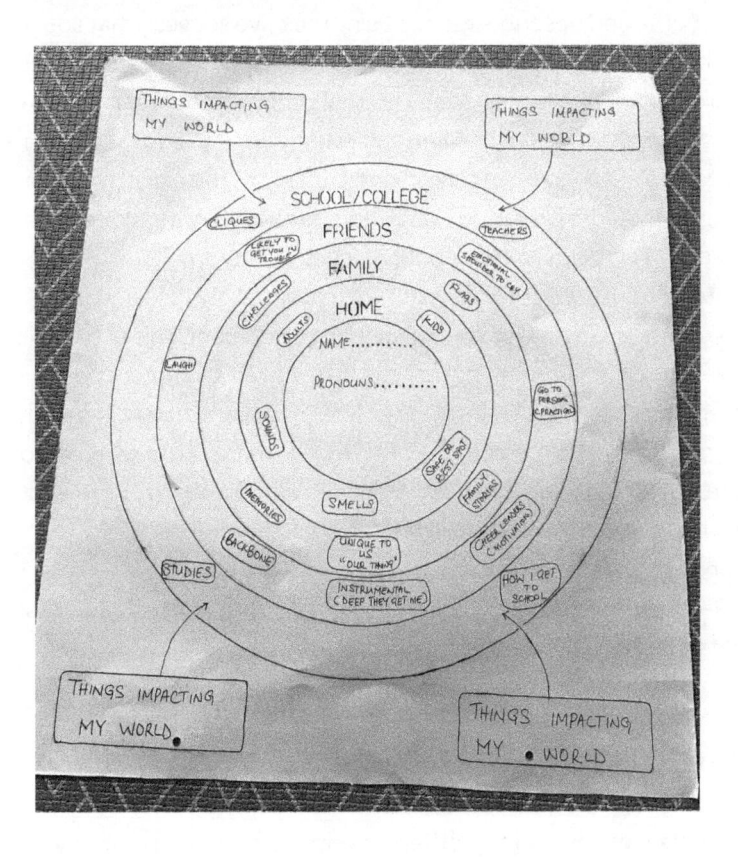

One of the circles is labelled 'friends', and the question prompts are based around the Cognitive Behavioural Therapy (CBT) theme of a backup team. As well as giving me a picture of their world and who is important to them, this helps me to identify what support network they have in place already. Another circle is 'family', and my question prompts help me to understand their identity. I am a London-based therapist; London is full of diversity and people from different backgrounds, so my questions help me bring race into the therapeutic conversation. This is why I include a couple of flag templates for them to tell me about their heritage. The circle labelled 'home' gives an insight into their home life, and this is the circle for which I tend to change the question prompts the most. For example, I find different ways to ask about the client's favourite place in the home, as everyone's home circumstances are different. With clients for whom it is appropriate, I use the opportunity to introduce a Mindfulness activity in this circle. I simply ask them to close their eyes and picture themselves in their home or their favourite spot in the home and describe it to me using their five senses: what sounds do they hear, what smells are around, what do they like to eat, what does it feel like and what can they see? The final circle is 'school and college', as I predominantly work with children and young people in education, although this can be changed to suit the client. Outside of the circle, I have arrows facing towards the circle and I label those arrows 'things that are impacting my world'. This helps me talk about reasons for therapy.

I tend to use this resource in the first or second session, along with icebreakers and establishing a counselling agreement. This usually fills the whole session. It's something that can be revisited at different points in the therapy, particularly at the end to see what has changed. It works really well in person as you can use a range of art mediums to form a creative collage piece, but I discovered that it also transfers well to working online – you can send it as something for the client to do before the session or you can work on one or two circles per session.

Resource ideas include pipe cleaners, felt paper, wool/string, lolly sticks, paints, cardboard, magazine cut-outs.

REFLECTIONS

- Be curious and try different approaches to assessing your clients' goals, needs and progress. What suits your client here?
- Consider using number scales to help reflect on where the client is in the moment.
- Help clients to recognize their journey by keeping a creative log of any shifts, skills and tools that they have found helpful throughout the process.

Chapter 5

Creative Activities and Interventions

In this chapter, we will explore ways that we can integrate creativity into our counselling sessions, from working with art, to poetry, to mosaics. You will also hear from some members of our Creative Counsellors Community who are passionate about integrating creativity into their work and offer examples of some of their favourite interventions.

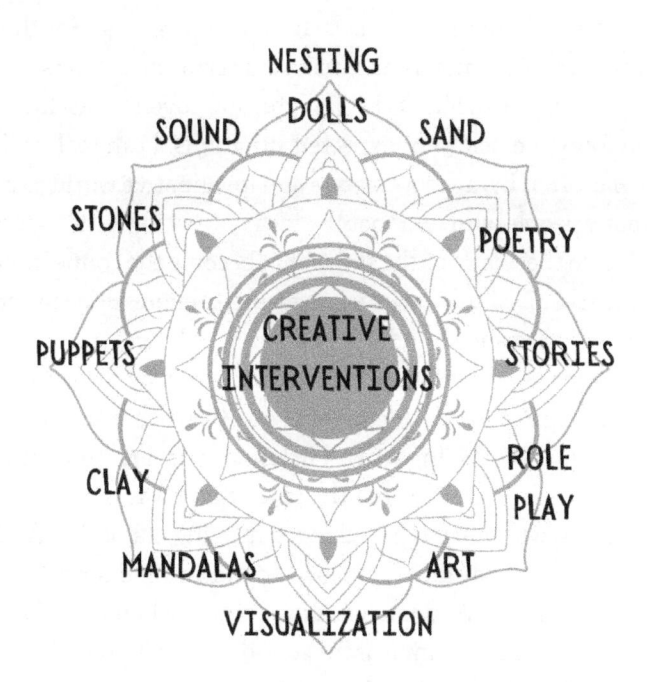

NESTING DOLLS
SOUND *SAND*
STONES
POETRY
PUPPETS **CREATIVE INTERVENTIONS** *STORIES*
CLAY *ROLE PLAY*
MANDALAS *ART*
VISUALIZATION

WORKING CREATIVELY WITH SOUND IN THE COUNSELLING ROOM

> **PRACTICE:** What songs or sounds would you include in your life's timeline? Starting from as far back as you can remember, can you connect with sound in particular stages of your life?

Cultures and people all over the world have historically recognized the power of sound as a healing, celebratory, connecting, storytelling and spiritual practice. We see evidence of this in our cultural stories, folklore, music and art.

In Zimbabwe, the Shona people use the mbira, which is a thumb piano made of 24 keys. They sing and play melodies to heal people from mental and physical illness, and this is a part of their connection to their ancestors. Hawaiians play songs (mele) to bring balance and health to the body and enable the flow of mana (life force) to rise. In Australia, the Aboriginal didgeridoo (yidaki) is estimated to be over 40,000 years old, and the healing rituals used there are said to have healed broken bones, illnesses and mental struggles.

My earliest sound memory is that of a TV series in South Africa called *Liewe Heksie*, which is an Afrikaans term that means 'Beloved Little Witch' in English. She was a forgetful and adventurous little witch and often found herself in unexpected situations. I can really relate to this, as I was often living in a creative and imaginative world as a child.

For many people who find that the idea of working with sound resonates, it is also the words of the songs that become the connector or the healer, and in counselling work we can facilitate expression through the use of music, lyrics and sound. When I think of lyrics, another significant sound memory that comes to mind is framed by the song 'Today' by The Smashing Pumpkins. I remember exactly where I was, what I was doing and how I was feeling when I listened to it. I remember having my shoes up on the dashboard of the truck that I was travelling in and singing happily, with my hand ducking and diving out of the window as we travelled. It was a day filled with love, friendship and connection, and the words of this song resonate with me on days when I feel full of joy.

Finally, I can recall an unpleasant sound memory from when I lived in Botswana. We lived within a small, gated mining community and every year the local authority would pay men to walk the streets and kill any stray cats, dogs and animals that were loose. I remember clearly the note my mom placed in the window to show that our animals were safe, and I have a deep sense of a feeling of unease, tightness and sadness in my stomach. I can still hear the sounds of gunshots ringing out and the accompanying smell and taste of gunpowder in the air as I clung to my two dogs and over 30 cats and kittens that we'd rescued. We were a safe haven for animals, and even though I can connect most intensely to the sounds of gunfire, I can also connect warmly to the sounds the cats made when Mom would stand at the kitchen door, singing for them to come home. The trees would begin to rattle, and it would rain cats and kittens each and every night as Mom, the Pied Piper, herded them in to eat.

We are surrounded by sound, and not only do we hear it, but we can taste it, feel it and sense it in different ways, too. When I hear the ocean and waves crashing on the shore, I can taste salty air and cheesy chips. This is because of what I associate with these sounds.

When I walk near to my home, there is an area of tall, swaying trees where I often go to sit and think. This area is full of life, movement and sound, and the trees are busy with nesting birds and a chorus of song.

I have a specific place that I like to sit when I visit there, because the sound is so clear and creates an echo through the trees. I like to close my eyes and tune in to the hypnotic tones that surround me, and when I am here, I feel 'tuned in', relaxed and at peace. I believe that we all tune in to different sounds and that these create different feelings and experiences in our inner worlds. I wrote this poem a few years ago, and it shares my personal experience with sound.

I AM
When I am with the birds, *I am tuned in*
When I am with the ocean, *I am healed*
When I am with the wind, *I am energised*
When I am with the rain, *I am renewed*
When I am with the snow, *I am at peace*
When I am with the drum, *I am a warrior*
When I am with the river, *I am in flow*
When I am with the silence, *I am connected*

Taking a moment to create an I AM poem with clients can be a beautifully expressive way to support them to make their own connections with sound.

Incorporating Sound within Other Creative Interventions by Masha Bennett

Masha Bennett, a Creative Trauma Psychotherapist and Trainer, shares her tips on incorporating sound within other creative interventions.

I specialize in Integrative Sandplay Therapy and Sound Healing, and love to combine these two modalities, but here I would like to offer some tips on incorporating sound with any form of Creative Therapy or counselling. You can usually do this with minimal equipment, but in case you might like to invest in a few musical/sound healing instruments, I will give a list of suggestions below.

Sound can have a profound effect on our nervous system. It can stimulate activity of the vagus nerve and trigger a powerful relaxation response; it may have a soothing effect on the amygdala – our 'emergency control centre' – and defuse the impulse of fight–flight–freeze; it may help lower the production of the stress hormone, cortisol, and enhance release of the 'feel-good' hormones, endorphins; application of sound can result in those pleasant tingling sensations known as Autonomous Sensory Meridian Response (ASMR); and when used skilfully and with therapeutic intent, sound can create powerful shifts in our emotions and cognitions.

I will describe three simple ways to incorporate sound with other creative methods.

- Using sound to facilitate *grounding and emotional regulation*.
- Incorporating sound as an *integral part* of client's creation/expression.
- Adding sound to the client's creation as *a healing agent*.

Grounding and Self-Regulation with Sound

You can use these simple techniques at the start of the session or at any point when the client – or you, the practitioner! – is feeling ungrounded or dysregulated.

- ✪ *Humming* – Demonstrate humming on a low note first, and then invite the client to join in. Get the client to notice where they feel the humming sensation in their body. Repeat a long, low hum together at least three times.
- ✪ *Drumming* – Invite the client to beat a drum, if possible, whilst stamping their feet on the floor to the beat. Optional: Suggest beating the drum at approximately 60 beats per minute/1 beat per second; this can help to promote an optimal heart rate, as the heartbeat will tend to synchronize with the beat of the drum.
- ✪ *Listening* – Invite the client simply to listen to the sound of a singing bowl or a bell until they no longer hear it. Ring the bowl or bell up to three times if necessary, each time allowing the sound to peter out gradually until neither you nor the client can hear it.

Sound as Part of the Client's Creation

As the client creates their sand tray, draws, paints, moulds, makes a puppet, etc., they may spontaneously create sounds (humming, sighing, laughing, groaning, etc.). Or they may mention music or certain types of sound when they talk about their work. For example, 'The bird is singing in the tree,' 'I feel a buzzing in my ears as I look at this picture,' 'A song came to mind when I was making this,' 'It is almost like I can hear the drumbeat.'

If the client is spontaneously creating their own sounds as they work, you could reflect on that and encourage them to do it consciously, For example, 'I am noticing you were humming a tune as you were creating/drawing etc... I wonder if that tune is part of this sand tray [or drawing, other creative work, etc.]?'.

The response may be 'No', and the client may not believe that there is any relevance of the tune or hum, in which case we can leave it at that.

If the response is 'Yes', and/or the client mentions sounds as they talked about their creation, you can invite them to consciously and intentionally add the sound to their work, for example: hum or sing the tune (or, if they prefer, find the tune online and play it through their phone); give a few 'pretend' sighs or groans on purpose; or use a musical instrument or another prop to create a sound.

If the client does not mention or represent aspects of sound or music in their creation (sand tray, art, clay, etc.), you may still intuitively feel that the addition of sound could be helpful. If you are sure that it would be helpful and appropriate, you can ask a question, such as, 'If there were a sound to go with your sand tray, drawing, clay creation, etc., what would it be?' or 'If there were a song to go with your sand tray, etc., what would it be?'.

The client may or may not want you to join in with making the sound or may wish for you to be the person to deliver the sound to their creation, so you could give them the option to invite you to participate, for example, 'Would you like to create this sound by yourself, or would you like me to join in?'. It is important to ensure that the client does not feel they have to include you as a polite gesture.

Invite the client to experiment with the positioning of the source of the sound (i.e., their mouth, the instrument, the phone playing a song) in relation to their creative piece – the distance and direction the sound is applied from may be significant.

Caution: Be careful if the client refers to a 'scream' or 'wail' in their description of sounds pertinent to their creative piece – whilst it is essential to acknowledge and validate this, it may *not* be safe or appropriate to encourage the client to actually scream or wail at full volume during the session, depending on the environment in which you work, your relationship with the client, the stage of their healing journey and your ability to contain the level of hyperarousal that may accompany such vocal expression. If the client does express a need to scream, it may be safer to invite them to do it at a much-reduced volume, unless you are absolutely confident in your capacity to contain and hold the client with the full intensity of their suffering expressed vocally, and your working space is adequately soundproofed and private to preserve confidentiality.

Sending Healing to the Client's Creation

Sometimes, there is no indication that sound forms 'part' of the client's creation. However, it is possible that adding the sound as a healing agent can still be of benefit. For example, 'I wonder, what type of sound (or song), if any, would be healing for your sand tray/drawing/clay creation? Would you like to add it?'.

As with using sound as part of the client's creation, the client may choose to send the healing sound themselves or may ask you to do it as well. Again, the distance and positioning of the source of the sound may be important.

Allow the client to decide on the length of time that their creation will receive the healing sound – it may be seconds, a minute, 10 minutes or longer. If they stop quickly, ask, 'Does this feel enough, or would this sand tray/drawing like some more of this healing sound?'.

If you work in an outcome-focused way, you may want to ask the client what difference they have noticed in their creative piece, or in their being, following the application of sound. For example, 'What's happening now? What's different?'. The client may or may not want to make changes to their creation after the sound has been added – let them do whatever feels right.

Useful Instruments to Have in the Therapy Room

Frame drum (ideally two so that both of you can play simultaneously if needed, or a larger drum you can use together, such as a 'Gathering Drum'), rain stick, ocean drum, thunder stick, chimes, singing bowl (ideally hand- rather than machine-made), wooden guiro ('croaking frog'), bell, shakers and rattles.

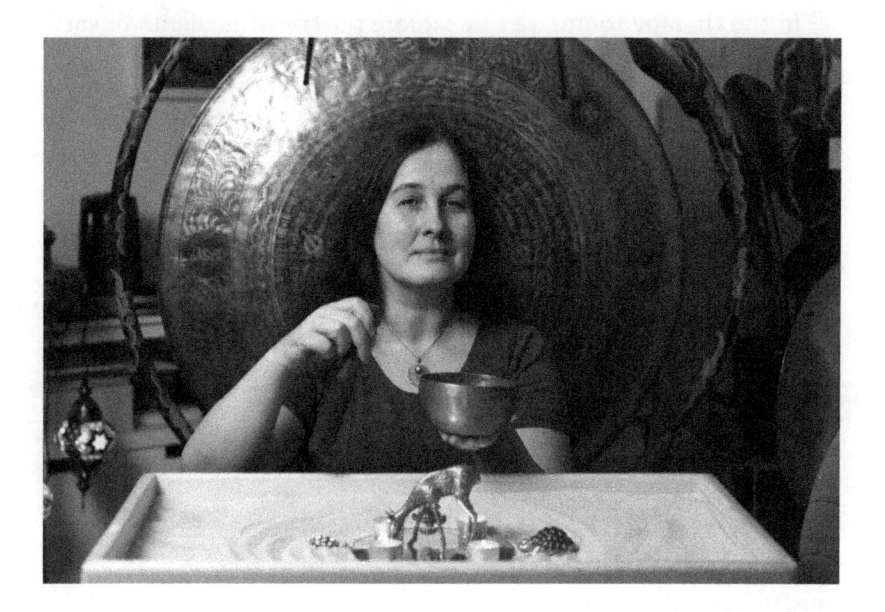

> **KEY POINT:** Sound offers us another layer of creativity to enhance Creative Counselling interventions. Be playful and try incorporating elements of sound into different exercises and approaches.

POETRY AS A CREATIVE INTERVENTION

I have always been drawn to poetry as a healing tool. I love how when I write, I can get lost in the words and they don't need to make sense. I will often work in an unstructured free-flowing way, adopting a curious and non-judgemental approach to writing. You could often find me, as a teen, sitting out on the boulders in the bay watching how the sea would crash in and retreat. I would write imaginatively about what might be happening in the depths of the ocean – what life we had yet to understand and what worlds we had yet to discover. In my own recovery as a survivor of sexual violence, I tapped into my creative side, and through the self-therapeutic use of poetry and writing, I was able to express and give a voice to my experiences, feelings and emotions. I would always carry a notebook with me so that I could doodle my words when they came up for me.

In the therapy room, we can explore poetry with clients in various ways and I would like to share three of my favourite approaches with you.

The Three-Line Poem

This simple check-in poem invites clients to create three simple lines that they can relate to in the moment to connect with their feelings and emotions.

EXAMPLE

> When my voice is taken
> When my soul is shaken
> Then all appears deeply lost

Mindful Poetry

This way of writing invites clients to tune in to their surroundings and write lines that describe what they are seeing, sensing and feeling in the present moment without structure or thought. This offers us an in-the-moment insight into what the client may be experiencing.

EXAMPLE

> My heart skips a beat
> The river flows
> That tree is tall
> The sun shines on me
> My mind is full of words
> I think of her face
> My heart skips a beat
> I feel sadness
> The wind is cool
> I want to cry
> The sand is warm under my feet

PRACTICE: Take some time to tune in to your environment. Write a few lines of mindful poetry that represents your experience right now.

Focusing on a Theme

In this way of working, we can support clients to explore a specific topic. This could be a person, a pet, a place or anything else that is important. It gives space and time for clients to reflect on and make sense of something that feels significant for them.

EXAMPLE

> His hands were cold
> His eyes were kind
> His smile was gentle
> His heart was wild
> His embrace was comforting
> His words were strong
> His life taken too early
> His memory lives on

In these three simple examples of how to integrate poetry into Creative Counselling work, I have focused on ways that feel less intimidating for clients. I would typically help clients when needed to create a mind map to connect with words, images, colours or anything else that can support their writings and then we would work together. I am as involved as the client directs me to be. At the end of the session, clients will often take their poetry home, but in some cases, we may burn the paper, flush it away or even create another creative exercise around this. I would encourage you to work in any way that feels good for you and your client. There is no right or wrong way to create poetry.

INCORPORATING ROLE PLAY IN THE COUNSELLING ROOM

I remember the first time that I was asked to role play in my counselling training. I was terrified and completely struck with fear. I remember thinking, 'How can I pretend to be someone else with someone else's problems and not look totally ridiculous doing this?'. If someone had told me then that some years later I would be embracing role play in my counselling practice, while wrapped in scarves and with a puppet in my hand, I would have never believed this. Now, I see the magic of role play in our community work, training, group therapy and one-to-one work.

Role play empowers clients to play out their situations and emotions. They get to explore what they are experiencing in different voices, from different angles and in different ways. I have witnessed profound healing, growth and transformation for clients through role play.

Simply inviting a client to embody the body language that they are experiencing from a partner can bring new insight to a situation. Playing out a difficult conversation that a client is fearful of, or even expressing feelings that don't feel safe to be expressed anywhere else with the use of puppets, can create some distance from overwhelming emotions that feel too heavy to hold.

In a recent peer-support training practice, I was partnered with Rebecca, who embodied the behaviours and mannerisms of someone with whom I had experienced a difficult conversation. She repeated some of the phrases that I had experienced from this person back to me, and I was overcome with emotion. This felt raw and real, and it helped me to make sense of why I had carried some unease and pressure for some time. With new insight, I was able to accept and release those judgements and offer myself compassion for what I had experienced.

> **KEY POINT:** Clients often experience big shifts in awareness of their relationships to others when you incorporate role play into your counselling work. They often get to see or feel things from a whole new perspective.

Working with Poems, Embodiment and Role Play by Rebecca Watson

I am excited to welcome Rebecca Watson, Dramatherapist, as she shares her thoughts around working with poems, embodiment and role play.

Embodiment and role work are an integral part of my dramatherapy practice. I have found, from years of practising as a dramatherapist, that this activity is effective with a range of clients from all different backgrounds. The gentle approach and use of laddering helps the clients to connect and engage with this activity in a safe and non-threatening way. This activity works well as a group or individually.

I select a variety of poems with different themes and characters; around ten for a group and five for individual therapy. I print or hand write them on different coloured paper, and invite the clients to read the poems in silence and select one they connect with.

I ask the clients to find a space in the room and read the poem to themselves in silence at first and then out loud. I encourage the clients to move around the space, speaking the poem out loud – using different tones and volume, repeating lines that resonate with them.

I invite the clients to memorize the line from the poem that most resonates with them and create a still image (using their bodies) of how that line makes them feel. The clients are invited to say the line out loud while holding the still image for at least one minute, repeating the line as many times as they need.

Repetition in dramatherapy helps to create containment. I have found with this particular activity that repeating lines from the poem helps the client to connect safely with the unconscious and heighten the potential therapeutic understanding.

Repetition allows for transformations to occur. One of the benefits of repeating words or sentences is the relaxation it produces in the body, allowing for blocks to be removed and for us to tap into a higher state of consciousness.

If this activity is being used in a group, I allow for other members of the group to step out one by one and witness the repetition of words and still images. Playing the role of witness can offer a different perspective; the client may not realize that they are tensing their shoulders or that their facial expression looks sad or longing. The witness may connect with the image personally, which can allow for further growth and development in their own process.

Role work is the final step of this activity, I feel it is important to assess whether the group is ready for role work. What are the group dynamics? Do they feel safe?

There are various dramatherapy techniques you could use when facilitating role work. You could choose hot seating, mask work, script writing, improvisation, and movement and sound.

De-roling is a crucial part of role work; this brings the awareness back to the present – to the here and now. In doing so, it allows the client to reflect on their experience.

I like to offer the client the opportunity to lightly pat down their bodies, starting from their heads and moving down towards their toes. For young people, I offer the metaphor of shaking off little droplets of water. I then ask the client to say their name out loud, reconnecting again with themselves.

I allow time to process and share any life drama connections. For individual therapy, this will be around 15 minutes; for groups I allow 25 minutes. However, I always gauge the response from the activity and if more time is needed, I allow for this, to ensure that the activity and any connections made are contained.

I have felt very privileged to witness this activity in therapy; it is powerful and moving. This activity has appeared advantageous to clients when words are not enough – connecting with their bodies and allowing the unconscious to manifest through embodiment and role.

CREATIVE ART INTERVENTIONS IN COUNSELLING

Art in counselling offers clients a way to express their emotions, feelings, desires, beliefs, thoughts, experiences and dreams. This can be facilitated in many different forms and can include anything and everything that helps them to communicate therapeutically, often without the need for words. In counselling, we might support clients to express their emotions through collage, painting, drawing, doodling, graffiti and sketching; we are only limited by our imagination and our resources.

We all have parts of us that we can find hard to verbalize. These parts can be fundamental to a client's recovery, so offering a space to explore through art can often lead to some of the most beautiful and inspiring moments in their therapy journey.

Some of the simplest ways to facilitate art in the counselling room include sketching, drawing and doodling.

I have always had a love for doodling and have published a series of 'CBT doodling' books that explore different therapeutic themes and invite readers to connect with a message and doodle away! I always have doodling ideas, worksheets and prompts ready for clients to use to explore what might be on their minds, and I have witnessed just how powerful this very simple approach can be.

Creative Doodling

To doodle is simply to daydream or move fluidly on paper. When it comes to counselling work, if clients are anxious about art, I will often facilitate the beginnings of a doodle, assisting them to find a starting point. We may doodle a simple creature based on what they are bringing into the room or even start with word doodles and play with shapes from there.

I always like to encourage the use of a boundary, just like a sand tray offers a safe space to work within; we can facilitate this with a simple outline to work within. I often talk about this with clients, setting the tone that this doodle page is their safe space to explore whatever may be appearing during the session. We can work with doodling in a mindful way, connecting the body, the mind and the emotions. This approach is great for first-timers or anyone nervous about being creative.

Free-Flow Doodling

This exercise works beautifully with a black waterproof marker, A3 paper and watercolour paints. I tend to introduce this exercise with uplifting and empowering themes like 'Celebrate Me', 'My Strengths', 'My Dreams and Goals' or 'Loved Ones', as we invite clients to spend a while really focusing on this creation. I have also worked with this method to explore loss, anxiety, relationships and abuse, but I would recommend that you have a very safe relationship with your client and that there is a definite purpose for working in this way. For example, clients have asked to work with doodles around these themes, as they have previously doodled in our sessions and found it to be helpful. With this in mind, they know what to expect already and can make an informed choice to keep themselves safe during the session.

Begin by assisting your client to think of a theme that would support them in this exercise. Invite your client to close their eyes and keep their pen on the paper. Begin with helping them to connect with the paper and the materials and to really set the intent for allowing a space to be non-judgemental and curious. Invite your client to keep their eyes closed and to begin moving their pen across the page, keeping the connection with the paper throughout. Once you have facilitated this for around a minute or so, your client will have created a series of lines, squiggles and shapes on their page. Next, invite your client to create an outline on their page to create their boundary all around their doodle. This can be any shape and size that they feel drawn to, and there is no right way or wrong way to create this. Once they have their boundary, invite the client to begin to fill each space within the shapes with other doodle lines, shapes and colours. Watercolours are great for this exercise, as they dry in different unique forms and tones throughout the page. Once you've assisted your client to add their colours, invite them to add any words that feel important in the moment. Now you will have a whole landscape of patterns, colours, words and shapes to explore together. Take some time to reflect on what has been created, and if it feels right, you may like to invite your client to give their creation a title.

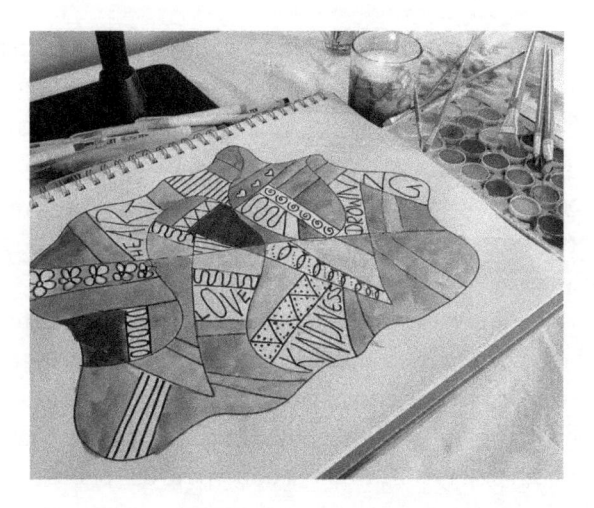

PRACTICE: Take some time to experience creative doodling for yourself. What comes up for you? What colours are you drawn to? What words?

Memory Boards by Evie Sharpe

Evie Sharpe, an Integrative Creative Counsellor, Coach and Mindfulness Mentor, shares her love of working with memory boards.

One of my favourite interventions to introduce with clients is memory boards, as they are so versatile and lend themselves to being used in such a multitude of ways. Memory boards are visual boards portraying people, places, times, emotions or challenges your client may have faced through life and can help them to gain a deeper understanding or new perspective on where they have been or where they want to go next. For thousands of years, people have used art to tell their stories, from the ancient drawings on the walls of caves portraying timelines and memories, to more recent creative art. Visual stories are so powerful and can tell us so much about a person and their way of life. Utilizing this powerful creative intervention in the counselling room can really deepen your client's understanding around the work they are doing as they process each memory and each part of their story.

Memories are such a fundamental part of who we are: knowing how to get out of bed in the morning, how to brush your teeth or make breakfast, how to drive a car, where you work, the names of the people around you and your own name, age and identity; remembering your child's first step or the smell of your mother's perfume; understanding your fears or reactions. Everything we do throughout our day relies on either already knowing and recalling information or the ability to read/learn new information and recall that when necessary, and yet how often do we really think about how our memory works, how we process and retrieve information and what we can do to preserve the memories we hold closest to us so that we are able to call upon them when we want to remember?

Memory boards are usually created using pin or cork boards to which you attach your memory items to build a picture or story portraying the memories you are working with. For items that cannot be pinned, I like to use little see-through bags or wrapping of some kind, such as ribbon or natural string, to create something pinnable. Another option is to use photos of the items, which can be pinned to the board. If your client does not have access to pin or cork boards, you can invite them to create their piece using big pieces of card or other materials they may have available.

Strengths Board

I also like to work with a strengths board – a board that pieces together all the times in your client's life when they have been proud of themselves, times when they have overcome challenges or difficult situations, times when they have shifted something in their life, and times when they have shown strength and determination. They can fill their board with as many memories as they can recall using photos, cards, certificates, words torn from magazines or newspapers, gifts they've been given, words they've written on paper or art they've created. Then they can start to look for more – that goal they got as a young child on the field with their friends, that swimming race they won, the courage to leave a partner who wasn't right for them, turning up for their exams even though they were so nervous, that session in the gym in which they ran further then they had before, that time they stood up for themselves and spoke out about something they felt passionate about and all the times they have had to handle or overcome something in their life. Invite your client to fill their board with all the incredible moments in their life that remind them of how strong they can be and of those times that they have experienced a positive shift. If appropriate, you may like to suggest to your client that they talk to friends and family about memories they may have of the times they have seen them display strength and overcome challenges or obstacles in their life and add these to the strengths board (if this feels right for the work you are doing with them). You may invite your client to take a moment to reflect on the positive emotions they felt in those moments and then suggest that they write those feelings down on paper or sticky notes to highlight those positive thoughts and emotions. Your client may like to pin these to the board too and fill the board with all their strength-building characteristics. When it's ready, invite your client to stand back and take a minute to really appreciate those strengths and skills, perhaps visualizing and breathing into those and really allowing this to integrate at a deeper level.

A Challenge Board – Whose Voice Is That?

Another empowering exercise is creating a board on 'Whose Voice Is That?', looking at all the limits your client has placed on themselves, all the things they have told themselves they can't do or aren't good enough for and all the times they fear they have 'failed' or not achieved the things they set out to achieve. Invite your client to use photos, bits from magazines or books, paint, collage or any other items they have that recall situations in which they have internalized that they are not good enough or other negative self-talk and to pin those to their board. Beginning to explore the board with your client, inviting them to start to question where those thoughts and voices came from. What age were they when these situations occurred? What skills have they learned since then? Are they still the same person now? Where in their body do they feel these emotions? What would they be doing if they did not have that negative self-talk? How are those beliefs limiting them? What self-talk would empower your client instead? What statements could they come up with that would make them feel good? What words could they begin to use to build their confidence? What would your client now like to say to that younger version of themselves? Can they offer themselves self-compassion? It is important to end this session with your client feeling empowered and able to begin to identify their negative self-talk so that they can begin to flip those thoughts and replace them with things that will help them to grow and move forward. You may invite your client to write down those positive statements, words or realizations and place them over the negative memories to begin to build a new picture of self-compassion and self-acceptance. Change takes time and can be challenging, but helping your client to understand where their limiting belief system has come from and challenging those thoughts and feelings to grow better, stronger roots can be such a rewarding exercise in self-awareness and self-empowerment.

There are so many ways in which memory boards can be used – remembering beautiful moments with parent/carers who are working through empty-nest syndrome, remembering loved ones your clients have lost or pets no longer with them, exploring different aspects of their personality or gaining a deeper understanding around how they behave in their relationships, exploring their boundaries, exploring their wild side, reconnecting to their inner child, exploring addiction or exploring their connection to nature. Your client may choose to keep their memory boards as they are or may feel more comfortable taking them apart again before the end of the session. I usually invite my clients to take a photo of their work if they would like to so that they can reflect on the piece if they choose.

Memory boards can be a very deep and powerful piece of work, and we always need to ensure the client is feeling safe and grounded before leaving the session.

The journey to self-discovery is one of the greatest journeys we can go on, and memory boards are a powerful tool to use for yourselves, as counsellors, too. When we are ready and willing to look at ourselves and explore our innermost thoughts, fears and emotions, we can choose to begin to see ourselves with the self-compassion and self-acknowledgement we deserve. As with all creative interventions, it is important to have practised memory boards for yourself before using them with clients, as you are working directly with personal memories, emotions and core beliefs.

Have fun!

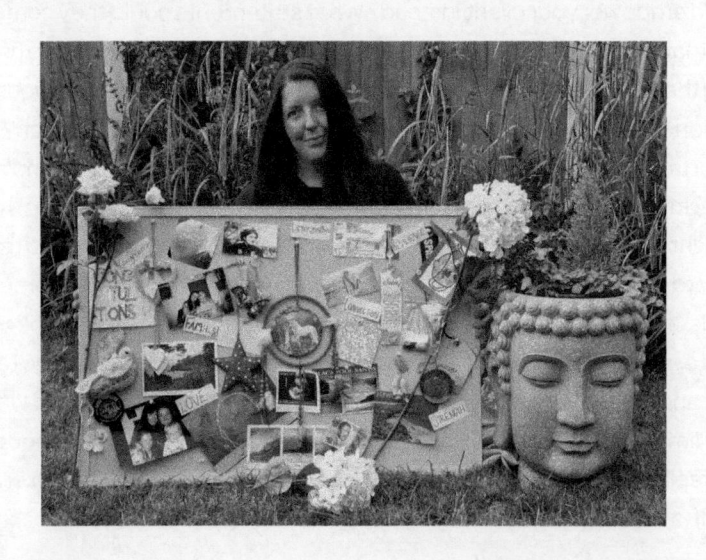

PRACTICE: Is there a theme that you would like to explore with memory boards? Take some time to collect materials that could represent this theme. Create your board and then reflect on the process. What was this like for you? Would you like to give your board a title?

My Creative Pet Intervention by Caroline Peacock

Caroline Peacock, an accredited Play and Creative Arts Therapist, shares her 'My Creative Pet' Intervention with us.

This is such a versatile way to connect to our subconscious, drawing out our wishes and needs in a gentle way. The client will only be made aware, by themselves, about what they are ready to receive at a given time. Clients can repeat the exercise periodically and see how it evolves with them and supports them to grow within the process of their healing.

1. Invite your client to gather materials in nature and add any additional materials that will help to bring this intervention to life, for example clay, buttons, feathers, material, etc.
2. Guide your client to imagine a safe place in nature (you might like to help the client with a guided meditation for added relaxation if needed).
3. Guide your client to visualize your their pet as it makes its way towards them, knowing that it is there to support them .
4. Explore using creative questioning like:
   - Where do they live and what is their dwelling? You could work with photographs, paintings and other materials.
   - What sounds can you hear around you when you are with your pet and what sounds do they make? Use a stethoscope to hear your own heartbeat – do you both share a heartbeat? What noises do they make? Do they sing, talk, whistle, etc.?
   - What do they feel like? Warm or cold? (If you have materials around you, help your client to invoke what it may feel like and to connect on a sensory level.)
   - What do they smell like? (Having some samples of different smells in your room can be helpful if this helps your client, e.g., fruit, herbs, essential oils.)

- What do they eat?
- When do they prefer to be awake?
5. Collect materials around you and invite your client to begin creating their 3D pet.
6. Ask your client to allow their pet to come to life, and if it feels right, you could work with some role play here, for example 'Ask your pet what its name is.'
7. If your client needs prompts you could ask these questions.
    - What message does your pet have to bring you?
    - What message do you have for your pet?
    - What does your pet need?
    - How can you help your pet?
8. Take a moment to reflect on the exercise with your client and remind them that their creative pet is always there for them.

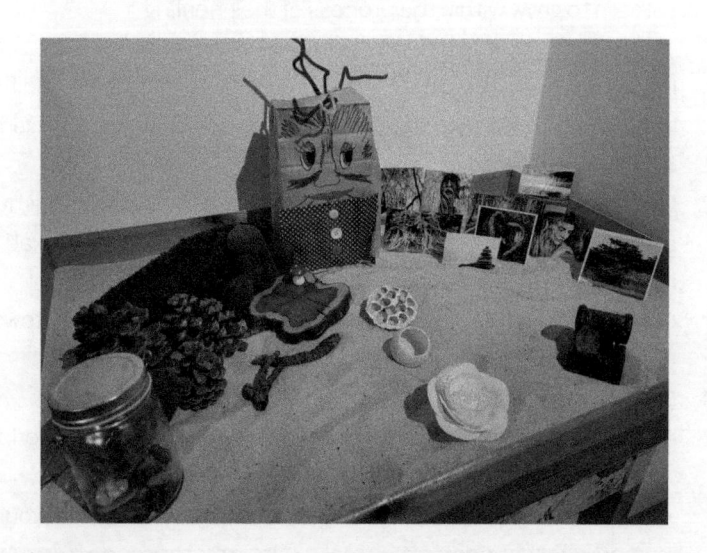

CREATIVE THERAPEUTIC JOURNALING

In 2018, we developed our first Creative Counsellors Online Course, and this introduced 50 Creative Therapeutic Journaling prompts and themes for counsellors. This has been one of our most popular courses, and we have welcomed members from 99 different countries to join us and journal.

Journaling offers us such a rich and diverse therapeutic approach to exploring anything and everything that clients bring into the room. This is also a wonderfully nurturing way to promote our own practitioner self-care. All you need to take part is something to create in and a load of varying materials that you are drawn to working with. It's as simple as that!

We asked our course members to share what they valued most about our creative journaling course and there were some common themes among the answers.

- As you are creating in a closed book space, this feels private, secure and different to creating a piece of art that is on show.
- It's so versatile and you can explore anything that you are drawn to focusing on or nothing in particular at all, meaning you can create just to create or create with purpose.
- It becomes addictive! Many of our community members have continued on with their journaling practice and produced incredibly beautiful and emotive books filled with life experiences.

The best way to explore facilitating creative journaling for your clients is to experience it yourself first. Take some time to create around these prompts. This could be using art, writing, poetry, collage or anything else that you are drawn to.

- Challenge yourself to write five positive things about something that you dislike.
- Create something to represent who you are when you are being your true self and who you are when you are being your false self. What feeds into each of these?
- Doodle something that represents your safe place. Where is this? Who else is there with you?
- Think about someone you admire or look up to. What are the qualities that you most admire about this person?

Expressive Visual Journaling by Honorata Chorąży-Przybysz

Honorata Chorąży-Przybysz, a qualified Therapeutic Arts Practitioner and Integrative Counsellor, shares how we can incorporate 'expressive visual journaling' into our work with clients.

Since I was a child, I have been attracted to the power of visual books. Whether that be a notebook filled with sketches, a scrapbook with photos or a fully painted book. There is something about the way that pages can open up possibilities of imagination and creativity. It's no surprise that my own favourite therapeutic tool is expressive visual journaling. The term is very broad and basically serves as an umbrella for an unlimited way of working in any type of book. There are many names and variations that can be examples of visual journaling: scrapbook, collaged book, art journal, sketchbook, smash book, visual diary, creative diary and so on. I believe that expressive visual journaling is a term for not limiting or labelling what we do – quite the opposite: *it is an unlimited source of creative, therapeutic and visual possibilities.*

The one thing that is the same about all the different styles of books and journals is that they take the form of a book: they have pages and a cover. Humans have a very symbolic attachment to books. In childhood, we hear stories read out to us, and later, we learn to write in books or journals. We may begin keeping a diary or maybe even a secret diary where we pour our thoughts and feelings on to the paper. Cultures are full of books with special meaning. From mythology, to the Bible, to 'forbidden books', they are present in many layers of our conscious and unconscious life. For therapeutic purposes, working in books can be kept private, personal and intimate. A book, unlike a canvas, doesn't have to go on display; it can be buried on a shelf or kept under a pillow. Books can be taken with us on the journey and become our daily companion. A book is a safe space to explore feelings, show vulnerabilities and use arts in a way that is not going to be displayed for judgement. When I mention keeping an expressive visual journal to clients who are working with arts therapeutically, I am very often (if not always!) met with sparkling eyes of inspiration and a willingness to start. Somehow, we do know intuitively that creating in this way will be kept in our hands, and we will be able to take ourselves on the journey of healing and self-exploration. Let's see how!

What Type of Book?

You can use any book; there is no need to invest in expensive materials. I work with clients using discarded textbooks, old comic books, simple plain sketchbooks or art journals. Textbooks are great as they provide a layer of text that can be incorporated into mixed-media work. Some clients have a specific book that they are ready to use for a visual journal. I have also worked with discarded guest or visitor books and empty old-fashioned photo albums. The choice is the client's, and there are as many personal preferences as there are people. Any book can be used, because by covering pages with gesso or white acrylic paint, or even gluing a few pages together (when the pages are really thin), we can create a solid ground to work on with many different art media.

Techniques – an Ocean of Creative Possibilities

Any art media can be used in expressive visual journaling. This is a space for freedom and exploration, for no right or wrong, for a client to accept their own creative expression without any need to meet aesthetic standards. The most effective techniques and combinations that I can recommend from my practice are listed here.

- *Collage* – Images from magazines, scrap papers, daily items like tickets, leaves from the park, receipts from shopping, one's own photos or even pieces of fabric or lace. Anything can be glued on to pages with a good dose of PVA glue.
- *Mixed media* – Using additional art materials with collage in a free, bold, colourful way. Acrylic paints and watercolours can be used for collage backgrounds and applied to pages directly. Pens, markers and pastels will give beautiful lines on top of the collages.
- *Writing and visual imagery* – A journal is a great place to write with a free-flow approach and to add imagery or even cover the writing.
- *Abstracts based on emotional responses to colour* – Use pages as canvases without needing them to look a certain way. Feelings can be easily translated into colours or brush strokes, and paint can even be applied with fingers. A journal provides an opportunity to play with colours and releasing emotional states.

Some Therapeutic Interventions for Expressive Visual Journaling

These therapeutic interventions are particularly effective when used with expressive visual journaling.

- *Exploration of Self and Inner Child* – The journal can be dedicated to that one subject (The Book of Self). Using themes around identity and life story, as well as working with childhood photos in the book, will provide a great tool for powerful exploration.
- *Life Story* – The journal can be divided into chapters and each one can symbolize a different chapter in life, which can be explored with visual techniques of collage or abstract.
- *Emotional Daily Diary* – Keeping a reflective diary that combines visual and writing techniques can become a rich and unlimited source of self-expression. Drawing, painting and gluing collage can all be included on the page where writing also takes place.

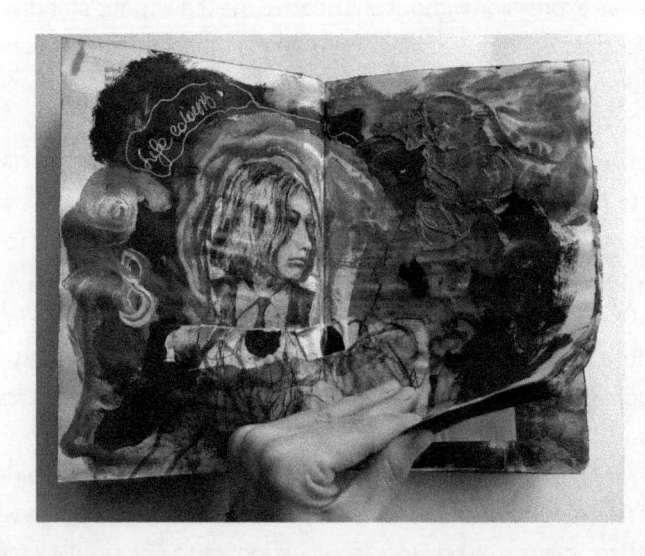

WORKING CREATIVELY WITH MANDALAS

Mandalas incorporate geometric designs that often begin at a centre point and work outwards. The intricate designs and hypnotic patterns can often work with the unconscious mind in magical ways in counselling work. Mandalas have been cherished for many years in traditions, cultures and religions across the world. Mandala is actually a Sanskrit word for 'circle' and is significant in Hindu and Buddhist cultures. As a creative tool, a mandala is often used as a meditation or focusing tool due to the intricate designs.

We find mandala shapes in so many everyday examples around us, from the iris of the eye, to a flower as it's opening, to sacred stone circles like Stonehenge, to dream catchers. The circular shapes can be filled with any designs, colours and patterns, and this creates endless opportunities to explore.

When I introduce working with mandalas to clients, I will often introduce the concept as representing both the external universe (what is around us), including relationships that we have with our environment, people, places and things, and the internal universe (what is within us), representing our beliefs, emotions, feelings and spirituality. We can focus on either or both as we are creating, and clients can often spend many sessions working with one mandala shape and the presenting themes that accompany it.

> **KEY POINT:** Mandalas are one of our most flexible tools, as we can work with these to explore many aspects of a client's life from childhood, to addictions, to anxiety and everything in between.

Mandala Worksheets by Denise Richards

Denise Richards, a Creative CBT Therapist, shares her love for working with mandala worksheets in the counselling room.

I first started using mandalas as a personal activity, a way for me to manage my own anxiety. After realizing the benefits mandalas can have, I enrolled in a class to learn how to create them for myself and later decided to incorporate them into counselling sessions as a means of greater expression and helping quieten a busy, occupied mind – one full of the never-ending thoughts, worries and concerns associated with anxiety.

I realized I could use mandalas as an alternative to traditional worksheets, as I found some clients I worked with didn't have the necessary literacy skills to be able to complete certain homework tasks (which are traditionally a part of CBT therapy) due to varying circumstances. On occasion, some clients shared that they felt stressed when thinking about completing worksheets; I wanted to remove that stress from the counselling room yet still use the tools I was trained in. Mandalas have become an alternative tool that enables clients to express their thoughts, feelings, emotions and behaviours in place of certain established worksheets.

Sometimes, the best way for a client to convey how they are feeling in sessions is through creativity rather than using words. I was finding that clients were adopting the mandala when I suggested it to them, and I decided to incorporate it more into my work as a result. This allowed my clients to be more relaxed and present in their sessions.

Mandalas can be used for specific purposes, which makes them such a useful and creative tool in the counselling room. They are extremely versatile, as they can be used in relation to many issues, such as grief, anxiety, stress, self-esteem, mood tracking, self-care, self-harm and anywhere else your imagination takes you.

In terms of anxiety, mandalas bring a wide variety of benefits to the client. They help promote relaxation and can reduce stress, helping to release tension. Colouring and focusing on the mandala will allow the brain to have some rest and relaxation, which for some may be much needed. When a person concentrates hard enough, they can experience the mental state of 'flow' – being completely immersed in a feeling of energized focus and concentration – allowing them to be more present and experience things in the here and now.

The very nature of creating a mandala is therapeutic, and it can be as simple or as complex a process as you wish. You can use a compass and protractor; you can draw around circular shapes; you can draw completely freehand. The client has the choice to work in whichever way they choose. However, if they wish to take a little time to create their mandala, they can use an array of materials, including charcoal, coloured pencils, watercolours, etc. The goal is to engage with the mandala exercise. Encourage the client to follow their instinct and to express themselves with whatever words, symbols or patterns feel natural to them at the time.

Colour is an optional element for mandalas, but it can take the client's work to a whole new level. This can be something you explore together to understand why the client chose specific colours and the emotions behind those colours. The symbolic nature of blue, for instance, can be seen to represent sadness and could be an entryway into further exploration of feelings and emotions. You can also explore the symbols used in the mandala. If there are repeating designs, you could take the opportunity to explore their meaning and how they work throughout the piece.

The mandala shown is one of my most recent designs and is a representation of my own anxiety. The straight lines in the inner and outer circles tend to represent structure and foundations, a sense of security for me to look at whenever my anxiety gets too much. The wavy lines in the outer circle help relax and calm me and take me back to when I was concentrating on making them in the first place. The beach was a heavy inspiration to me for this one, and it is a place I always end up going to as it helps to ground and calm me whenever my anxiety gets too much. The circles drawn under the wavy lines were directly inspired by a pebble beach and the tide lapping up and down across the shore. The pattern in the middle was something I did unconsciously until I interpreted it to be a pattern of a seashell I saw whilst walking along the beach. Finally, the mandala as a whole made me feel safe and held, the circles acting like a life ring.

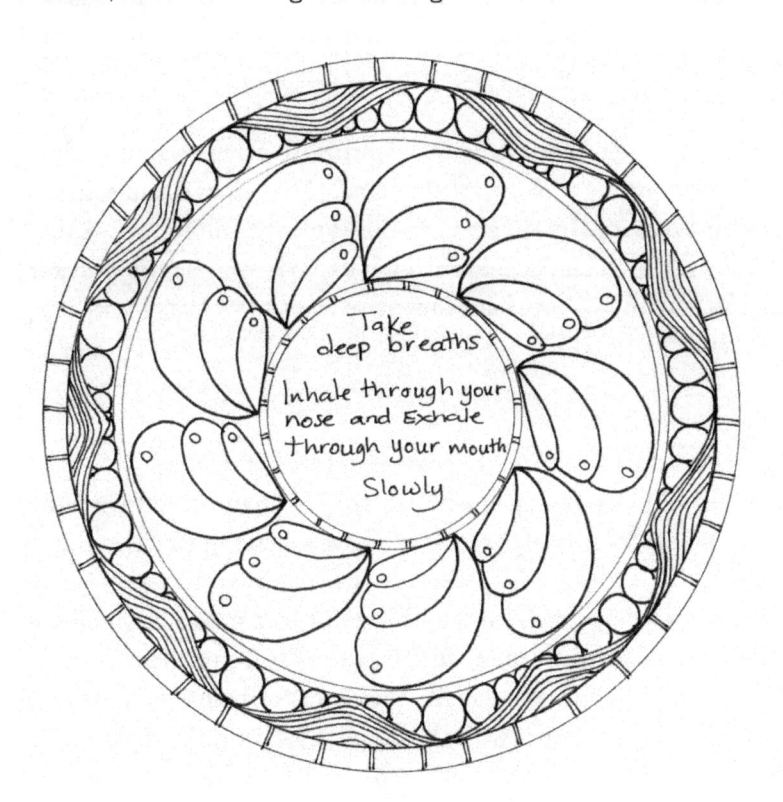

WORKING CREATIVELY WITH CLAY IN THE COUNSELLING ROOM

When I lived in Devon, I would visit a pottery studio where we could create and paint our own ceramics, and my son loved this. I have warm memories of sipping tea and chatting with other visitors while we created and painted. When I look back now, I can see how therapeutic this was even though we did not fully realize it at the time. This simple but wonderful act of working with natural, earthing materials in our hands, creating whatever shapes came to mind and doing this unconsciously while we talked with each other – there was a magic in this!

I went on to facilitate outdoor play sessions in woodlands with children and young people, and clay would find its way into almost every session as we created tree warriors, hidey holes, gremlins, wands and doorways for the trees. Even the most 'unengaged' young people would find a way to engage through clay, getting lost in the process.

We know that clay was used in Ancient Egypt and Ancient Greece, and in medieval times. It's likely that clay was used to line baskets and water carriers to enable easier transport of water, and we find evidence of art creations made from clay in many cultures from tools to symbols to pottery.

In the counselling room, we can work with clay in a multitude of ways, incorporating tools, symbols, hands, feet, elbows and sound.

In our Working Creatively with Clay online training, we explore how to work with clay safely through experiential hands-on exercises and learning. One of our favourite ways to work is by creating clay bowls.

Clay Bowls

Clay bowls act as a natural container, and this can offer a safe space to work within. The theme of a bowl is that of nurturing and holding, and psychologically, I feel that this can have a calming effect on clients when working with anxiety, loss and other painful presenting issues.

To create a clay bowl, I invite the client to create a clay ball and then to make hole with their thumb in the centre of the clay. Then, with the thumb in the hole, I invite the client to pinch the sides of the clay bowl while rotating it with the other hand, working their way up from the bottom. They can create some additional height in the bowl by pinching and gently pulling the clay as they move upwards. It can help to keep adding small amounts of water when needed.

Once the bowl is created, I invite clients to add anything that they would like to the bowl to create permanent patterns, maybe some petals, stones, paint or anything else they are drawn to. When it is dry, it can act as a container for the work, and we can add words, symbols, images or anything else that the client would like to work with.

I have found this to be a particularly useful exercise for supporting trauma survivors.

> **KEY POINT:** Clay is a naturally grounding earth element. It offers the client a way to mould their feelings and experiences into something visual, which can then be explored.

Working with Metaphor and Visualization Through Clay by Cara Cramp

Cara Cramp, a Child and Adolescent Creative Arts Therapist, shares that her favourite creative intervention in the therapy room is working with metaphor and visualization through clay.

Working with clay in therapy can bring into conscious awareness that which has been unconscious. It can activate forgotten memories and sensations and provoke big emotions – but in a safe and containing way. It can be used to express and process non-verbal ideas and concepts in a way that verbalizing sometimes cannot. Using clay can be both messy and neat, and the great thing is that the client can choose which it is going to be.

Clay can be an introduction to safe touch, and through clay, clients can explore touching their own hands as well as those of their therapist. Clay is like a living metaphor: it is from the earth and so can symbolize life itself; it can be what we make it. Clay is usually cold and shapeless when we first take it out of the packet but as we begin to mould and project into it, it takes our energies and begins to warm. These are the reasons why I love to use clay in therapy with clients.

For this exercise, we are working with metaphor and visualization. It looks at what is stopping a client from moving forward in either their recovery or emotional journey and how they can reframe that into something that will help them rather than sabotage their progress. They can do the exercise with their eyes open or closed, whichever they prefer.

We will be using sculpting and hand-building for this exercise, but it can also be adapted for using clay on a potter's wheel. Using clay on a wheel gives a vastly different experience, but for some clients, using a potter's wheel can be a transforming and enlightening experience. It can be a chance for a client to get messy and it can be an opportunity, through the process of centring the clay on the wheel, for the client to gain mastery over the clay and at the same time visualize taking mastery over something in their own life.

> Therapist: What would your saboteur look like if it had a visual form? Use the clay to create this. Remember that we will not keep the clay in this form but use the same clay to create something that will assist you rather than hinder.

The client then creates a saboteur and describes what they have created.

The therapist then asks the client to squash their saboteur and encourages them to take ownership and autonomy over it to create a new visual form that is going to remind them that they can move forward and be successful.

In this example, the hammer represents the automatic negative thoughts in a client's head feeling like a hammer crushing her spirit and ability to listen to the truth about herself. They control her behaviours and keep her locked in the past. The candle holder reminds her she is free; she can use the candle as a Mindfulness tool when she wants to clear her head, focusing on the flame of the candle and how it moves. The saboteur has been changed and reformed into something that is positive for the client.

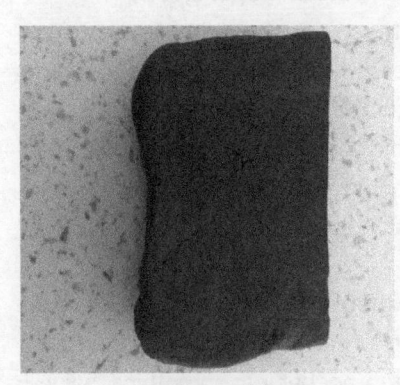

Initial piece of clay

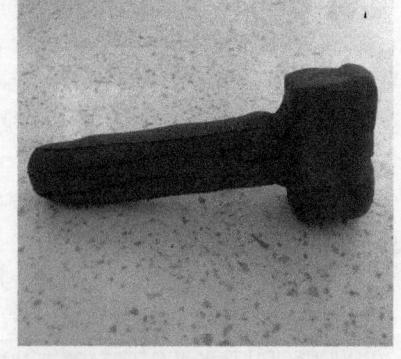

The saboteur takes the form of a hammer

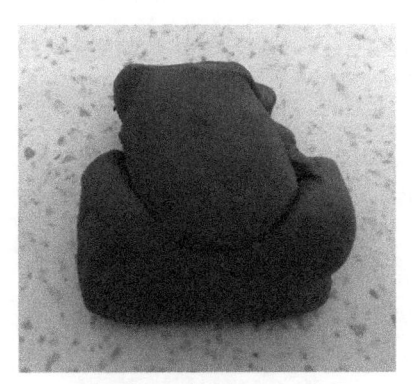

The saboteur has been crushed

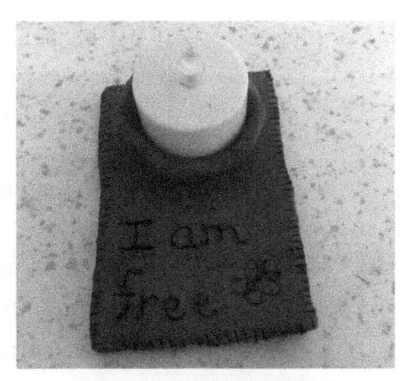

The same clay has been used to make a new form

⁓ Working Creatively with Mosaics and Ceramics by Rhiannon Davies

Rhiannon Davies, a Creative Integrative Counsellor, shares her love for working with mosaics in the counselling room.

I am very drawn to mosaic as a tool in my work with bereaved clients and those experiencing relationship problems.

In life, we have all broken something that has meant something special to us, and we have had our hearts broken. I love how the Japanese art of Kintsugi – kin (gold) tsugi (repair) – celebrates our broken pieces by gluing them back together to create something new and wonderful. So, when an object breaks, this does not mean it is no longer useful. Its breakages become its beautiful parts, and to me this symbolizes the essence of resilience.

Each of us should try to look at the parts of us that have broken, search for ways to cope with traumatic events in a positive way, learn from negative experiences, take the best from them and create growth; these experiences make each person unique, precious and valued. With this tool, it is possible to create true and unique works of art, each with its own story and beauty thanks to the unique cracks formed when the object breaks, as if they were wounds that leave different marks on each of us.

I would invite my client to do this exercise towards the penultimate session – to create a piece to represent their journey: accepting the reality of their loss, experiencing the pain of the loss, adjusting to the new environment without the lost person and engaging in the new reality.

I call this exercise 'The Seeds of Growth'.

A mosaic piece can be created from a variety of items: broken crockery, glass, shells, stones, jewellery, pictures, keys, etc., and items you may pick up from walks or holidays.

I use the following resources for this exercise:

- terracotta plant pots (pre-seal with PVA to make them less vulnerable to frost damage – they are not suitable for cold weather); alternatively, you could use jars to make candle holders
- PVA glue/silicone adhesive
- acrylic paint
- chalk or crayons
- plain/patterned pre-cut ceramic tiles
- client's choice of trinkets
- tile nippers
- gloves
- grout
- spatula
- cloths.

Method

1. Paint the pots with acrylic paint in the client's choice of colour before the session. Invite the client to think about a design that's as simple as possible – what items would they like to include on their pot/candle holder?
2. Invite the client to choose some squared tiles and place a continuous line of them along the top ring and bottom baseline. These are used to ground the client.
3. Invite the client to decide where the main trinket will be placed and the significant other pieces. They can draw in their locations.
4. Leading from the base upwards, invite the client to start placing the small irregular-shaped pieces in the design using a flexible knife and adhesive. Leave adequate gaps between the pieces – to represent the path of growth. Use different colours that may reflect the 'greyer', darker struggles: anger, depression, panic attacks, guilt, shame, flashbacks, an awareness of painful experiences. Place in trinkets

that represent things that helped: shells from a walk on the beach, a colourful stone to represent a friend, a piece of costume jewellery, a coin.

Creating can be cathartic. Clients may deflect or resist. Observe the process. Make statements of encouragement; increase the client's awareness; look at good things that have appeared through painful situations. Depending on the age group, use explanations to meet their level of cognitive development. Look at areas that they have had to work harder on and the lighter colours of enlightenment.

5. Once the pot has been filled, allow it to dry. Give the client the opportunity to grout their piece in the final session. Let them think about what they would like to put inside their pot. What type of flower, what fragrance candle, what colour will they choose? Does it evoke a memory of the person they have lost?
6. When the client takes their pot home, explain that it's best to allow it to dry off thoroughly for 48 hours and then give it a polish with a dry cloth. As the client polishes their pot, I might invite them to recognize how they are nurturing this symbol that they have created in recognition of the loved one they have lost.

While this way of creating mosaic can be used on a ceramic pot or glass jar, there is no end to the way we can use mosaics in therapy work, whether in collage form from old magazines on a blank piece of paper or in sand with pebbles or shells on a beach. Each client comes with their own story, their own personal interest. As a Creative Counsellor, I adapt my modality to suit each client.

WORKING CREATIVELY WITH PUPPETS

Working with puppets can enable clients to explore painful and difficult emotions at a safe distance by interacting and playing out scenes, roles and conversations. This often helps clients to bring a new awareness to a situation and to find new strategies and ways to deal with problems; this is especially powerful as a tool for empowering clients to 'try out' difficult conversations in real life.

Puppets come in a range of themes – from animals, to people, to imaginative characters – and you can find them in a range of sizes, from tiny finger puppets all the way up to full-grown life-like characters that sit on your knee. In my therapy room, I actually only have a small range of puppets, as one of my favourite ways to facilitate working with puppets is to create a puppet with the client. This creates a deeper and more personal connection for the client, and we can find out so much more about the presenting issue and how this is impacting on the client this way.

Conversational Puppets

This exercise is a great way to empower clients to recreate or experience a conversation that they would like to explore with someone else through the use of puppets. I have worked with clients to explore arguments with a partner, have a tricky conversation at work with a colleague, stand up to a bully, say goodbye to someone who passed and release anger towards perpetrators.

To create your own puppets with clients, all you need is a paper bag big enough to fit over the client's hand and some permanent markers, although sometimes we do end up creating wonderfully detailed characters using collage, paint and other magical bits we can find around the room.

Begin by inviting your client to think about the people or characters that they want to work with to represent those people. The client can then create the puppets by drawing these characters on the bags. Clients can add anything they want to their creations.

Once the puppets are created, your client may want to place them on both their hands, or they may want you to take on the role of one of the puppets. I would err on the side of caution when it comes to taking on the role of someone else. This can be tricky to manage because we often do not know enough about the 'other' person to accurately reflect their way of being, and, as therapists, we can find ourselves easily undermining clients or stepping into the 'fixing' role here. I much prefer to empower clients to take on both roles while I facilitate the conversation between them.

EXAMPLE

Counsellor: Can you introduce me to your puppets?

Client: On this hand, I have Jason, he's an annoying but loving big brother, and on this hand is Ellie, who is quite shy at home and doesn't really have a voice.

Counsellor: So, we have Jason and Ellie. Jason is an annoying but loving big brother and Ellie is shy and doesn't feel like she has a voice. I notice how much bigger Jason's eyes are than Ellie's and I'm curious about that.

Client: Jason has huge eyes as he is always looking over Ellie's shoulder and telling her what to do [the client places one puppet behind the other and over the shoulder]. Ellie has small ears and a small mouth because she is sick of hearing his voice all the time and wants to tell him to leave her alone but is scared to.

Counsellor: So, Jason has big eyes and a big mouth and tells Ellie what to do, and Ellie wants to tell him to leave her alone but feels scared. I'm wondering what she is scared about?

Client: Ellie is scared to hurt Jason's feelings because since their dad died, he has been taking care of everyone, and she knows that he is only trying to help and is missing his dad a lot. She just wants to tell him that she's okay and she doesn't need him constantly worrying about her.

Counsellor: This sounds like an important conversation and I wonder whether Ellie might like to try having this conversation now to see how it might feel?

Client: [Client faces the puppets towards each other] Jason, I love you, and I want to thank you for always being there for me and taking care of me. You are the best big brother anyone could ever wish for. I also want you to know that since Dad died, you have never stopped worrying about Mum and me, and I can see how exhausted you always are. You shout at us for every little thing, and you act like you know best for me. I'm an adult, and I know what I need and what's best for me. I want you to be my big brother again. The big brother who used to make me laugh and go to the movies with me and play pranks on me. I just want my big brother back because Dad isn't coming back, and I don't want to lose my big brother too!

> **KEY POINT:** Working with puppets can empower clients to play out conversations that they may find overwhelming or difficult to have in real life, giving them an opportunity to be heard, have their feelings validated and, in doing so, build confidence.

Worry Buddies by Tracy Dunning

Tracy Dunning, a Creative Counsellor, shares her passion for working with her homemade Worry Buddies in the counselling room.

I created a Worry Buddy to support a young client who was struggling to talk about their emotions both in sessions and at home. When I created this, I thought of the importance of the Buddy having a mouth to swallow up the client's worries, and I further adapted them to have pouches in their hands and to wear different hats. The different Worry Buddies can either 'hold the worry', 'eat the worry' or 'keep the worry under their hat', and clients can choose what feels right for them.

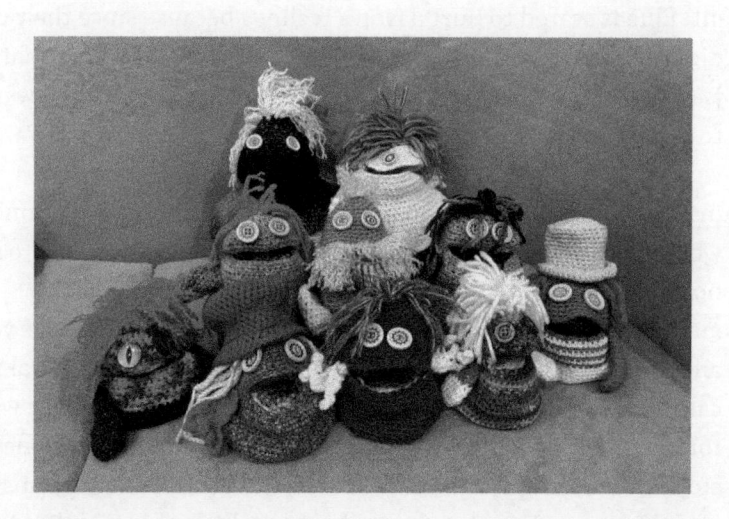

When working with these creatures, we can invite young people to take their Buddy home with them so that they feel able to express their worries at any time. Young people can bring their worries home with them and work with their Buddy or they can work with them on the go. Depending on the situation, and if it feels right, the counsellor, parent or carer can remove the worry from the Buddy so the child can relate to sharing the worry with someone and having a sense of this being 'swallowed up'. I have found this to be really helpful in the therapy room. At first, I created these to be used in counselling sessions, but as the word about my Worry Buddies spread, I found that parents began to use them, and friends and colleagues have done so too. I have also supported teachers to use them in the classroom setting, giving young people the opportunity to leave their worries at school at the end of the day.

Because all the creatures are different, this is a great tool for exploring our uniqueness and differences, as well as for opening up conversations around working with our worries and expressing them.

WORKING CREATIVELY WITH STONES IN THE COUNSELLING ROOM

Over the last few years, our Creative Counsellors Community members have fallen in love with stone painting, pebble mandalas and stone doodles for client work as well as self-care.

For years, I have been collecting stones from everywhere that I have visited, and I keep these in a basket under the sand tray. Clients are invited to work with the stones in their natural form or to paint them to represent people, feelings, emotions, hopes, dreams, goals or anything else that they are drawn to expressing.

Stones have their own energy; they are grounding, earthing, strong, often feel cool to hold, have quirky unique shapes and come in all sizes. They are a wonderful gift from nature to support clients' growth. There are many different ways that we can work therapeutically with stones, and I would love to share my personal top three with you!

Doodle Stones

This is a relaxing approach to doodling that offers clients something that they can take away with them as a grounding reminder.

1. Invite clients to choose a stone from your collection or to bring one with them to the session.
2. Using a permanent black marker (or any colour they prefer), invite your client to create free-flow doodle patterns all over the stone. Doodling on stones is extra fun, as they often have

unique shapes, rough edges, smooth parts and extraordinary shapes to navigate.
3. Invite your client to add colour to their doodles with acrylic paint pens in any way that they are drawn to.

I have found that clients experience relaxation, can explore painful themes more easily and often feel more grounded in the process while stone doodling.

As a self-care practice, I love to create these stone doodles for my own relaxation, and you may find this a beautiful way to connect with nature and create some creative space for you too.

Emotion Stones

Invite clients to choose a stone that represents an emotion they can connect with in the moment and add this emotion to the stone. They may like to choose a colour to represent that emotion or a word. They may like to add paint, collage, drawings or doodles to the stone. They may even like to keep this in its natural form without adding anything to the stone.

Collage Stones

I have been experimenting with various papers, tissues and glue and have found that we can create beautiful patterns on stones with collage. Working with paper can be less daunting for some clients who struggle with confidence around 'being creative', as it already has a pattern. The patterns are important too; I have created nautical-themed stones, African-themed stones, word stones and random patterns this way. As long as you use a collage glue and allow plenty of drying time, these can work out beautifully and become a great addition to your symbols collection for clients, too.

> **KEY POINT:** Stones are naturally grounding, therapeutic and versatile and are often palm sized; they can be a great addition to your counselling room.

Creative Ways to Work with Stones by Tara O'Kane

Tara O'Kane, a Creative, Person-Centred Counsellor, shares her favourite ways to work with stones in the counselling room.

'Choose an object that represents your journey on this course.' These words, used on the last day of my Level 2 training, sparked my interest in using creative tools in counselling. Since then, I have built up quite the selection of creative tools, but my favourite, without doubt, has got to be stones. Not only are they cheap (often free!) and easily transported, they are also so diverse in their look, their properties and their versatility. I have built up quite a collection from beaches, walks in the woods, garden centres and discount stores, in a variety of shapes, sizes and textures.

Person-Centred Counselling is classed as a talking therapy. The theory behind it is that the client knows what hurts and has the resources to heal and move forward by talking through their issues. However, there are occasions when clients find it difficult to articulate or verbalize exactly what it is they are feeling, when the words are too painful to say or when words alone do not do justice to what the client is going through. When this happens, my stones will make an appearance in the counselling room! The process of choosing stones is empowering for clients and having something physical that they can hold in their hand gives intangible emotions a sense of reality, which can be very validating.

Below, I share just a few of the ways I like to use stones with clients.

Exploring Relationships

I invite clients to choose stones to represent their family or people close to them and to place them either on the table or in a sand tray. It is so interesting watching the choices being made – how the client holds each stone and where they are placed in relation to each other. We then explore their choices, the features and placement of each stone (big, small, in the middle, out on its own), where the client is in the placement, how it feels looking at it and so on. It can bring a great deal of insight into their relationships that had previously sat in their subconscious.

Exploring Aspects of Self

Clients will sometimes choose a selection of stones to represent different parts of themselves. This could be aspects of their personality, their roles in life (father, son, husband, brother, friend, etc.) or the emotions they experience. It can be uncomfortable but incredibly powerful for the client, as they reveal parts of themselves that they have perhaps never shared or were even unaware of.

Mindful Grounding with Stones

Clients can become overwhelmed during sessions, and some find it difficult to regulate this feeling. I use stones to help clients bring themselves back into the present moment. I will invite them to choose a stone and to describe every detail of it as they are experiencing it: what it looks like and feels like. It is a nice way to end a session so that clients leave feeling calm and in the here and now.

Creating Story Stones

This is an intervention that I have used successfully with young people and adults alike. I have a selection of stones and ask the client to choose some to tell their story so far or what led them to this moment. The client then uses Posca pens to draw words, pictures, emotions or symbols as they place each stone down. I find this helps the client to truly see their journey, but they can see it from a distance, which means it can feel safer to explore it and tell their story. Some young people simply use colours for different parts of their story. Either way, the insight gained is often profound.

In all these exercises, clients may like to take a photograph of what they have created, and I encourage them to do this if they wish. Using stones as part of the client's process can help them to go to places that were previously inaccessible, gain new perspective and gently access the subconscious so that they can begin, or continue on, their healing journey.

Stones are such a powerful and versatile creative tool to use in counselling. I certainly would not be without mine.

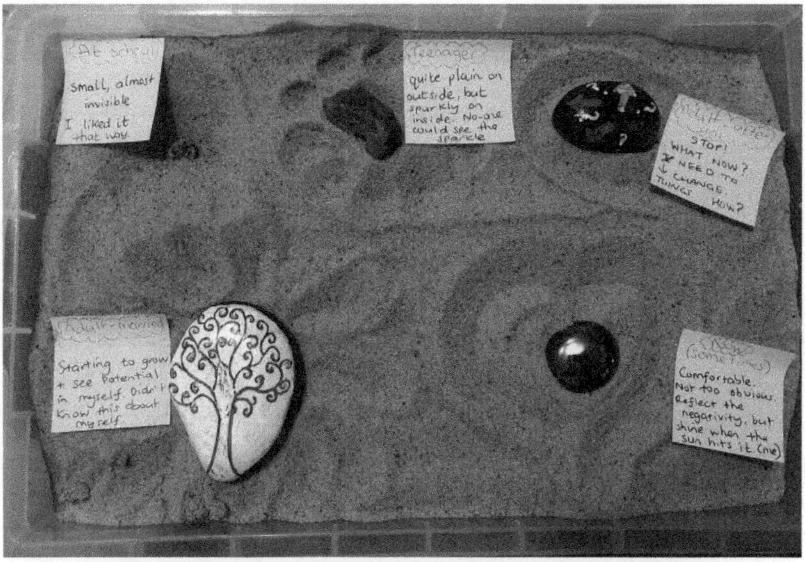
At school
small, almost invisible
I liked it that way.
Teenager
quite plain on outside, but sparkly on inside. No-one could see the sparkle
STOP! WHAT NOW? I NEED TO CHANGE THINGS HOW?
Starting to grow + see potential in myself. Didn't know this about myself
Now (Sometimes)
Comfortable. Not too obvious. Reflect the negativity, but shine when the sun hits it. (me)

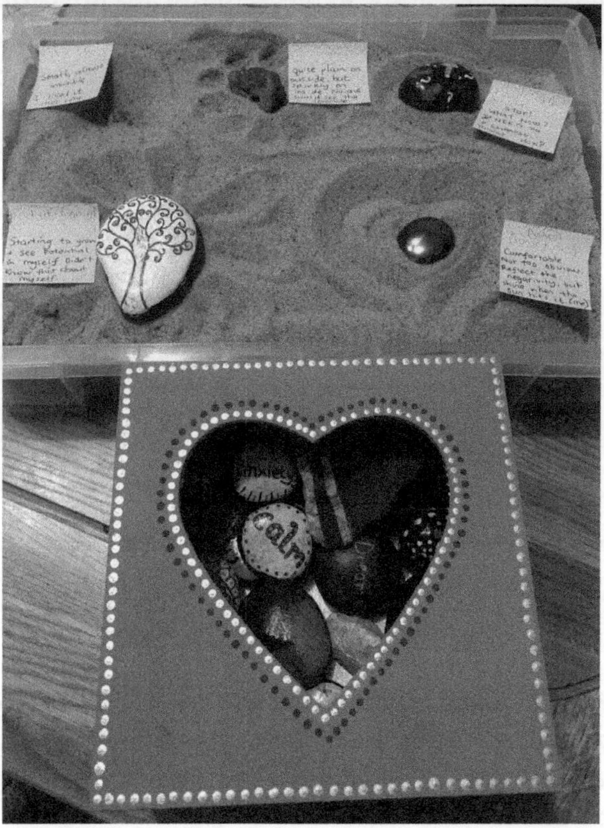
calm

WORKING WITH CREATIVE VISUALIZATION IN THE COUNSELLING ROOM

I remember reading my very first book on Creative Visualization, written by Shakti Gawain, many years ago and feeling this overwhelming sense of possibility and hope (Gawain 2016). I was learning for the first time how I could actually empower my mind to visualize what I wanted and to experience it as if it were real. I connected with how miraculous this could be as a tool for self-healing from my own traumatic past, and I wanted to learn as much as I could.

I began to write empowering visualizations for clients based on their hopes and dreams for their own healing, and I witnessed many incredible moments in which clients were able to release and to gain a new perspective while feeling safe, grounded and held.

Little did I know that I would be having my own profound shift a little while later while sitting in the third row at a live performance with Derren Brown. During this performance, I was guided through a Creative Visualization in which I took a walk on a beach to meet my most healthy, vibrant and empowered self. This experience was overwhelmingly peaceful and beautiful and empowered me to begin to heal through forgiveness. Seeing myself in this whole, healthy and healed way left me with a feeling of not being 'damaged' but being 'hurt', and the shift in this thinking released a deep-rooted sense of shame and heaviness that I had carried around with me, deeply buried in my gut like a boulder, for many years. I didn't see this broken person that I had visualized often, but rather someone who shone even though they felt hurt, and it felt good to recognize this healthy emotion so it could be released.

I believe that we have yet to scratch the surface when it comes to understanding Creative Visualization as a healing tool for working with trauma, and I continue to read as much as I can on this approach.

∼ Nature's Gift Creative Visualization by Lin Sharpe

Lin Sharpe, a Metaphysical Coach, Meditation, Mindfulness and Spiritual Teacher, shares her love for incorporating nature within her Creative Visualizations practice.

I believe that working with our imagination is one of the most powerful ways to support clients therapeutically to heal. I have witnessed this with many clients over the past 30 years of practice. When we work with our imagination, the brain does not know the difference between the real and the imagined, and we can harness this incredible gift within our work, helping clients to imagine a new way of being and feeling. Working in this way helps us to use visualization to create a positive experience or outcome for clients, and the more that we repeat this action, the more we are coaching the brain to accept this as possible. Possibility is like a seed that when nurtured and watered grows into hope, into self-belief and into wholeness. As we gain momentum by repeating this action, we create new neural pathways in the brain, and these become our new normal. Over the years, I have written many visualizations, which I now teach with my daughter Tanja in our Confident Hearts Creative Wellbeing Programmes, and I would love to share this Nature's Gift Visualization with you as a tool to support your clients.

This visualization has a number of therapeutic benefits that support clients to take time out and connect with their inner world. We go to nature for healing in many different ways and many clients will choose nature as one of their healing spaces, so this often feels like a natural and easy visualization to experience.

Some of our clients will tell us they do not have an imagination and, when this happens, we take the time to guide them gently, nurturing their confidence as they connect with this visualization. I have typed this visualization out word for word so that you can confidently offer this within your creative practice. My wish is that you and your clients, in working with this visualization, are able to experience the incredible gifts offered freely by mother nature, by your imagination, by your choice to find moments of gratitude, appreciation and peace, and by valuing yourselves and your lives – enhancing your life experiences always and in all ways.

Nature's Gift Visualization

Let's begin by taking some deep breaths, getting really comfortable, perhaps readjusting your position if you feel you would like to and uncrossing and relaxing your feet and arms.

Move your attention to your feet where they connect with the floor, feeling that solid anchoring with the floor, and where you are sitting on the chair and your back against the chair. Take some more deep breaths, really allowing the body to relax. Become aware of any tension that may have built up in the body and just give that permission to let go, coming gently into this now moment, aware of your breathing, aware of how your breathing moves your body, perhaps noticing how your abdomen rises as you breathe in and lowers as the air is released, the air moving in and out, in and out.

Now move your awareness to your heart, holding it for a moment on your physical heart, breathing gently into your heart, in and out, in and out.

Imagine you are walking along a path, strolling quietly along, being aware that you are going somewhere but you are not in a hurry to get there. As you look around you, you notice the tall trees lining the path moving and swaying with the breeze, the vibrant green plants in the undergrowth, the clear blue sky, the gentle, warm sun on your face and just a feeling of peace as you walk along. You hear the sounds all around you, perhaps trees moving with the breeze, the creaking of the branches, the rustling of the plants, the call of the birds as you allow your feet to take you on a gentle journey. As you move along, you feel safe and secure, knowing that this is *your* gentle journey and that nobody else can come into your space. This is your own personal space. You begin to feel a sense of letting go, of just being in this experience.

You become aware there are some fruit trees at the side of the path and you decide to choose one, breaking the delicious fruit off, and as you walk along, eating the fruit and appreciating it, you feel grateful for the gift of natural food that nature provides us with to energize and nourish our bodies.

As you round a corner, you see before you a meadow, a meadow that stretches out with a little stream running through it. There are tall mountains on the other side of the stream, trees, an array of vibrant colourful flowers spread out. You find yourself walking to the side of the stream where you notice a little clearing, a clearing with fine, green grass.

As you approach this clearing, although you are tempted to sit, you decide that you would like to taste some of that clear, pure water from the stream. Bending down, you cup your hand and you take some water, drinking it gently, marvelling at how nature provides water, that you can hydrate your body, the waters of life.

Now you decide you will settle down on the inviting, luscious grass so that you can look all around you and take this beautiful scene in through your senses. Getting comfortable on the grass, your attention is drawn to the stream in front of you as it gently meanders along its way, reminding you of how your life continues along each day, whether you are aware of it or not.

Sitting quietly at the water's edge, you notice now some leaves drifting gently along in the water. As you watch them, you see that one gets caught up against a rock as the other continues on its pathway. Yet, after a while, the leaf which has been blocked becomes free and sets off on its way again, whilst the other now finds itself momentarily stuck on the side of the bank, and you realize that this can be like life – where you sometimes get stuck with some challenge as life flows on, yet also realizing that after a while you free yourself and move once again into the flow of life.

Looking up, you become aware of some clouds drifting gently along in the blue sky, just as your own thoughts continuously drift through your mind until you give one your attention. Sometimes, the clouds come together to form a bigger cloud, just as your thoughts sometimes do. You remember that you can let those clouds just drift off again if you would like, without becoming attached to them, reminding yourself that they are just thoughts, or you may choose to focus on some of those thoughts.

You now find your attention drawn to a beautiful scent that fills the air and the glorious array of flowers comes into your awareness, nodding their heads in the gentle breeze. You marvel at the diversity of their vibrant colours and different types, and you are reminded of the rich diversity we find in life, of people, places, experiences, all of which come together to add to the whole picture of your life.

You become aware of the trees firmly rooted in the ground, their trunks strong, their branches reaching up to the sky, weathering the changes in the climate each day. You think of how you can be rooted firmly in your life's journey, building resilience and bending and moving with the storms in your life, yet ever reaching upwards to grow and evolve.

As you look across the stream, you look up at the mountains in the background, each uniquely standing serene and tall, pouring out their powerful energy to all. You reflect for a moment on how at this time in your life you can choose to make a choice to stand serene and tall in your own power, your own unique light, giving this freely to yourself as well as others.

As you sit there quietly breathing in the pure air, a butterfly lands on your hand and sits there gently, its little legs tickling your hand, and you find yourself amazed at the beauty of its form, wings with their perfect markings, delicate legs and feelers. As you take this in, it reminds you of how you can choose to take precious moments in your life and appreciate your own form, your own body, all the wonderful ways it has carried you and supported you in your life.

And as the butterfly now moves off in the breeze, you become aware of the pathway that brought you to the meadow and you ponder for a moment how you get to choose time and time again what pathways you will take in life, how each path leads you to a unique set of circumstances and how you can choose again and again if you would like a different outcome.

The soft, green grass underneath you now invites you to lie down. And you settle down comfortably, beginning to listen to all the sounds of nature, just allowing them to gently soothe you as you feel yourself dropping into a place of deeper relaxation. The warmth of the sun lulls your senses, the call of the birds in the background, the sounds of the running water, the movement of the trees in the breeze. You allow these sounds to move through you as you lie quietly on your grass carpet, and you become aware of a feeling of contentment and peace growing within you. You invite and open for a few moments to these gentle sounds and the majesty of nature as it offers its healing gifts deep inside your mind, your body and your feelings as you just lie quietly in the meadow for a few moments, being gently aware of the sounds all around you and of the feeling of relaxation, of peace, of quiet.

Now you become aware that it's time to return, and you gently stretch your body, sitting up and then rising to your feet, taking one more look around at the beautiful scene before you, knowing you can come back at any time you would like to.

Feeling relaxed and calm, grateful for all the gifts nature offers you, you begin your journey back, bringing all the feelings with you that you have gathered in this time with nature, all the gifts that you have received. Once again, you find yourself walking through the fruit trees with their abundance of delicious fruit as you follow the path bringing you back into your heart.

Taking some deep, even breaths, place your attention on your feet connecting with the ground, where you are sitting, your back against the chair.

As you come back in now, there is a quiet awareness within you, a feeling of gratitude for all the gifts that you have received from nature and knowing that at any time you can return to your sanctuary in the meadow. Taking a few moments and focusing on your Nature's Sanctuary, you can have those same feelings, healings and blessings.

Gently open your eyes, being aware of your environment, moving your hands and feet if you need to as you come fully back in.

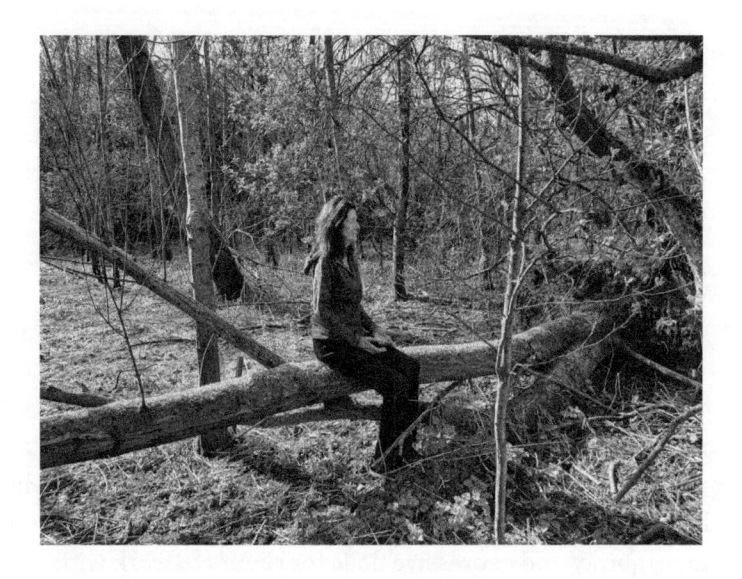

WORKING CREATIVELY WITH NESTING DOLLS IN THE COUNSELLING ROOM

Some historians believe that nesting dolls (matryoshka dolls) originated from Japan, however we know that Russian masters created hollow wooden easter egg holders and that the first set of matryoshka dolls appeared in Moscow in the 1890s. They have since become a popular collector's item around the world. Every year, when I travel to find artisan and festive Christmas markets, I find stalls lined with nesting dolls portraying Russian folk art in every shape, size and design that you can imagine.

These are also becoming more and more popular in the counselling room, and when I held my first Russian dolls training with a group of counsellors in 2018, we explored all the different ways that we could work with these to support clients. This remains a popular topic of discussion in our Creative Counsellors Community.

One of the things that we talk about a lot is the lack of diversity available in nesting dolls. Many clients don't connect with the traditional Russian folk style of artwork, so I felt it was important to share some ways that you can personalize nesting dolls to offer a more diverse range for clients to work with, as well as a few ways to work with them.

Chalk Dolls

Plain wooden dolls are great for painting with chalkboard paint. This offers clients a way to personalize their dolls as they work. Clients can write feelings, stories and words on their dolls or they can name them. When the work has finished, the dolls can be easily cleaned.

Collage Dolls

I was curious as to how plain wooden dolls would look if they were covered in a collage of different patterns and designs. I collected a variety of collage paper in different patterns and colours and started sticking these randomly across the dolls. The end result was strikingly beautiful and very original. I hadn't seen any dolls like these anywhere, and this quickly became a little obsession for me. I now have a range of unique, quirky and expressive dolls for clients to work with.

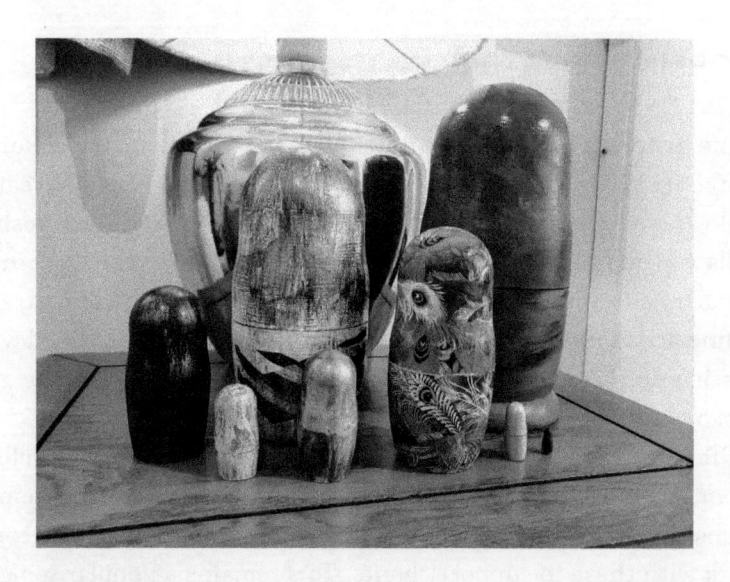

Painted Dolls

Many designs that you will find online are overcomplicated and too abstract, making it difficult for clients to fully connect with this as a metaphor or a symbol. Having some plain, painted dolls in block colours can be helpful. You can work with themes like 'What colour do you feel today?' or 'If his anger was a colour, what would it be?'.

Nesting Doll Timelines

These are a brilliant way to make sense of a client's history and memories in a visual way. Invite the client to pick different nesting dolls that resonate with different memories and times in their life. Invite them to notice how they are displayed and in what sizes. What could it mean for them if they picked the smallest doll to represent their married life and the biggest doll to represent the passing of a loved one? Could they be feeling insignificant in their relationship and did the pain of losing their loved one feel overwhelming and massive in their world at the time? These are only examples, and I would never assume or guess what it means for a client. Maybe they feel safe in their married life, and choosing the biggest doll for the passing of a loved one could represent survivor's guilt or a feeling of release from a burden. We can't know until the client opens the door for us and invites us into their world, from their frame of reference.

Hidden Messages

These nesting symbols are a great way to work with feelings and statements as they can be hidden away in the belly of the doll. You can invite your client to write a message or a statement and place this safely within the doll. Maybe an empowering new statement or a message of self-forgiveness. Maybe a series of gratitude messages or a poem broken down line by line and placed within each doll. The possibilities are endless here!

> **KEY POINT:** These symbols can easily be personalized by clients, making them an incredibly versatile tool to empower clients to take ownership of their symbols.

WORKING THERAPEUTICALLY WITH CHARACTERS, FAIRY TALES AND STORIES

PRACTICE: If you were a character in a film, what film would it be and what character would you be?

There are thousands of possible characters that we can work with therapeutically in the counselling room, including those from storybooks, movies, gaming and fairy tales, and real-life heroes and leaders.

As I am writing this book, I am also writing our brand-new Creative Counsellors training module in which we explore this in depth, navigating the curious world of characters. Maybe your client resonates with Alice as she is falling down the rabbit hole. Maybe they've had to lose their voice to be with the one they love, like Ariel. Maybe your client has a Jafar in their lives, controlling and manipulating their decisions. Perhaps they are fighting for their freedom, like Nelson Mandela, or struggle to be still, like Tigger.

There is a character, a story and a stage for every client dilemma that finds its way into your room, and we can utilize the power of characters to play these out with clients.

Who Am I?

You can invite clients to explore themselves and their different parts with characters. Which character represents their protective part? Which character represents their loyal part? Who are they when their needs are being met? Who are they when their needs aren't being met?

Relationships and People

Who does the client have in their world? Identify characters with whom the client resonates to describe different relationships in their world and look at how these characters interact with each other. Which character takes more than they give to the client? Which character is a grounding anchor for the client, and with which do they resonate most? When using symbols, pay attention to how the client places these and what their body language is displaying throughout.

Surviving Trauma

For some clients, finding the right words to express their trauma can be a massive challenge, and working with characters, fairy tales, stories and movies can bridge this gap and create a shared language that is helpful for the client.

EXAMPLE

Client: I just can't describe how evil she is!

Counsellor: I'm wondering, if she were a character in a movie, what character might she be?

Client: Medusa. Don't stay too long or you will turn to stone! She has no ability to feel or empathize with anyone else and the longer you stay with her the more you become frozen, numb and unable to feel!

WORKING THERAPEUTICALLY WITH SAND

Creating your story in the sand isn't just for children, it's most definitely for adults too!

Growing up, the whole beach was my sand tray, but I actually remember making circles with my feet and sitting inside them. At the time, I couldn't have known that I was creating a safe little boundary to be within so I could feel to heal my way through my pain. Looking back, I now understand more fully why I found my way barefoot to the sand each and every time I needed to just be.

Sand is made up of many different natural and weathered materials. The sand's components depend on the location, but the most common are silicon dioxide in the form of quartz crystal, feldspar and mica. Anyone who works with crystals and stones as a self-care tool will know what incredible energetic benefits we can gain from being with and around crystals. I believe that when I am facilitating a space for clients to work therapeutically in the sand, I am creating a healing space like no other.

There is something beautifully natural about placing your hands in a sand tray and making a connection with the sand as it falls through your fingers. A sense of 'in the momentness' or grounding. Some of the sand that we work with is over four billion years old, and it has been on a wild journey of life and death to find its way to us. Much of the sand that we work with also incorporates tiny particles of the exoskeletal remains of marine and animal life from our planet. When I am working with the energy in the tray, I like to take a moment to ground myself, to tune in and to offer gratitude to the earth and all of earth's creatures who journeyed with this sand. Oh, if sand could talk, the stories it might tell!

Clients will often not be aware of the power of the sand, so I take time to talk about the journey that it has taken to find its way into our room. Many clients find this tale incredible, and I watch as clients often begin to nurture the sand curiously with a childlike playfulness.

To Begin

I invite clients to connect with the sand and to ground themselves, taking some deep breaths as they move the sand between their fingers. Once grounded, I invite clients to begin to explore the symbols in the room and to find anything that they are drawn to bringing back to the sand. I watch and wait as the client places their symbols and begins to create their story in the sand.

Exploring

When I sense that the client has completed their tray, I will check in: 'I noticed that you seem to have finished creating your tray.' Then I will begin to follow our MBFI model to help clients to explore.

'I'm wondering if you can take a moment to connect with what you are experiencing right now as you look at your tray?' This facilitates clients to explore what is happening in their body. Once we have a connection, I may invite the client to share their tray with me: 'I'm wondering whether you may like to guide me through your tray?'

Clients are always ready to share and will only share what they feel comfortable with. If I am curious and something feels important, I may make some observations like, 'I notice that there is a shiny egg in the middle of your tray.' This will often nudge the client to keep exploring. I never interpret what I see, only notice and reflect. If I have a sense of saying something that is on the tip of my tongue, I will own this: 'I might be wrong, and this is my experience of what I see, and I'm sensing that the donkey struggles to face the snake and I'm a little curious about this.' We will explore together for as long as the client needs within our session time.

Endings

I invite the client to take a photo before they place their symbols in our endings tray so they can be cleaned and returned to their places in the room.

Many clients can feel a little dehydrated – in the way that your skin can dry out when being at the beach – so I offer a bottle of water and some advice to stay hydrated.

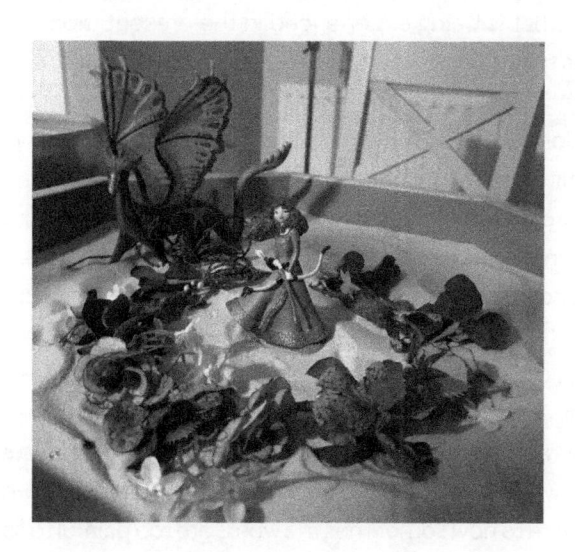

WORKING CREATIVELY WITH EMPTY CHAIR CARDS

~ The Empty Chair Cards by Yasmin Shaheen-Zaffar

Yasmin Shaheen-Zaffar shares her passion for working with the Empty Chair Cards that she has designed.

I have created digital cards that have been inspired by the Gestalt Empty Chair Technique, which have been invaluable since having to work online due to the COVID-19 pandemic. They are available to purchase on the Watoto Play website.[1]

You could say the Empty Chair Technique is one of the most popular exercises used in Gestalt therapy, often for 'unfinished business'. In the technique, a client sits across from an empty chair and is asked to imagine that someone else is sitting in that chair, for example a parent, ex-partner, ex-boss or known bully. Or they could imagine themselves or a part of themselves in the chair, for example their inner child, inner critic or shy self. The therapist then encourages the client to engage in a conversation with the

---

1   https://watotoplay.com/interactive-digital-therapy-resources/resources-category/the-empty-chair-cards-version-2021

imaginary person (or part of a person). As the conversation moves on, the client alternates roles, switching from one chair to the next accordingly.

I totally love this powerful Gestalt technique – it's all about bringing into awareness what is being experienced in the present moment. The only downside is that being asked to sit and talk to an imaginary person sat on an empty chair…well…errr…it can feel a little overwhelming, intimidating and confrontational. Not to mention sometimes a little, dare I say it, weird or strange. This led me to consider how could I find a gentler, less confrontational way of using the Empty Chair Technique. One that would open up conversation about the conscious but also the unconscious. And at the same time, not frighten or intimidate clients. And that's how I came up with the Empty Chair Cards.

Initially, I created the Empty Chair Cards as a warmup exercise to the Empty Chair Technique. But I have found that these cards have become a valuable therapy tool in their own right. Being dyslexic and a visual learner, I understand when clients feel disconnected to the spoken and written word, but I also relate to how sometimes the words are too painful to say outright.

I have found that these cards visually open up the conversation in a non-threatening manner. To begin with, a client flicks through the cards and picks one that they are drawn to or that resembles the issue or relationship they want to work on resolving. Or they pick the type of chair they would want the person with whom they have the 'unresolved business' to sit on; this leads to a conversation about the type of chair, why they have picked it and what that card means to them in relation to the relationship/issue they are working on.

Below are some ideas on how the cards can be used, but I am sure each therapist will find their own unique way of working with them. That's the magic of being a Creative Counsellor!

Give a Voice to Ruminating or Distorted Thoughts or Unfinished Business

- Ask the client to pick a card representing the person they want to talk to or the part of themselves that would sit on that chair.
- Explore why they are drawn to that particular card – what emotions or feelings are triggered in the now?

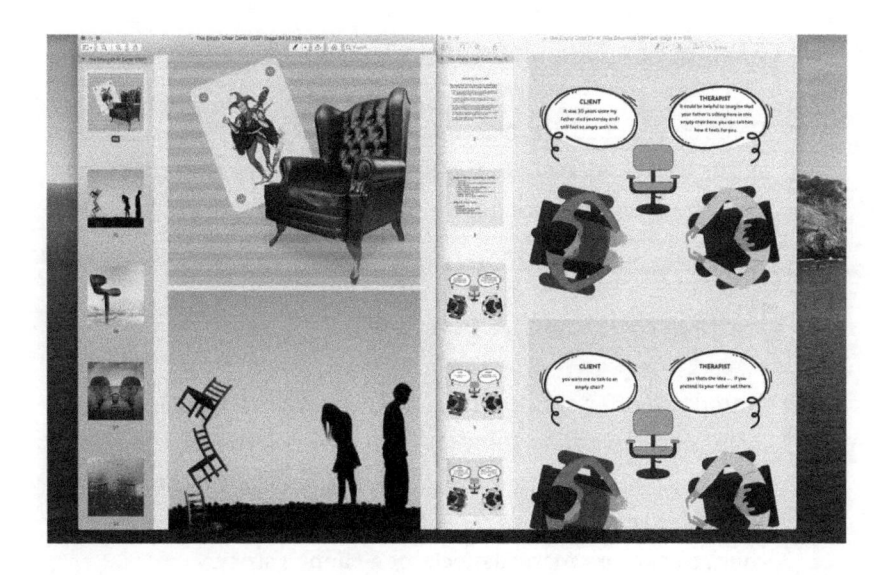

Bring the Unconscious to the Conscious

- ✸ Once the client has selected their card, we can help them to explore this and make sense of what the images and backgrounds mean for them. Would they pick a different card or background? The client can choose one chair on one card with a background of another card. Would they change the size of the chair, and would it be larger or smaller? Would they move it to a different position on the card?
- ✸ How does the card relate to the feelings brought up about the issue/person?

Visually See the Changes a Client Wants to Make

- ✸ The client picks two cards – one represents the relationship they currently have with themselves, the person they want to talk to or the 'unfinished business'. The second card represents the relationship they would like to have. Explore what change needs to take place for the relationship to move from the first card to the second card. How do they feel/think about both cards?

Help to Reflect on Their Journey in Therapy

- Cards can be used to evaluate and explore whether there has been a shift in the client's feelings, thoughts or behaviours. They can visually describe the therapy journey.

REFLECTIONS

- Sound can offer another layer to the work that you are doing.
- Role play can offer clients a fresh perspective on how they appear in the world and the relationships around them.
- Mandalas are one of our most flexible tools, as we can work with them to explore many aspects of a client's story.
- Many creative interventions offer naturally grounding and soothing elements, like clay and paint.
- Working with puppets can empower clients to play out conversations that they may otherwise find overwhelming or difficult in real life.
- Stones are naturally grounding, therapeutic and versatile and are often palm sized; they can be a great addition to your counselling room.

Chapter 6

Take Time to Reflect

In this chapter, we will explore the fifth element of our Create Circle Approach, supporting clients to take time to reflect as part of the process. We will explore the importance of this and how it can impact on the work.

EXPLORING REFLECTIVE PRACTICE

The way that we work as Creative Counsellors often creates a bridge between what is unconscious and conscious, so as we empower clients to creatively weave their stories and experiences into being, we must also hold space for clients to make sense of what they are experiencing in their own words, colours, shapes, lines, imagery and feelings. We need to be mindful of avoiding interpreting creations from our own perspective, as our perspectives are born out of our own life experiences, beliefs, relationships and experiences, and these won't necessarily be appropriate for our clients. Over the years, I have come to trust in the process and believe that our clients' unconscious minds know where they need to go and will only go where it feels safe to explore. I believe that our clients' bodies are wired to work in whatever ways they perceive are in their best interests, and their past experiences and how they have processed these fuel how we navigate our subconscious layers. With this belief and thinking, I feel safe to hold the room, to check in and ground when I sense this is needed and to facilitate a reflective space that, above all else, respects and holds the clients' experiencing in high esteem.

~ Working with Joy by Gaynor Rimmer

Here Gaynor Rimmer, a qualified Creative Counsellor and Hypnotherapist, shares her personal reflections around the theme of 'joy' with us.

Choosing a symbol for joy was a lot harder than I originally expected, and I had to dig deep and ask myself: 'What does joy actually mean to me?'. On reflection, I chose this palm-sized curious crystal family. Eight individual tiny crystals with little eyes and their own unique characteristics. As I began to create this, I realized that each one represented one of my grandchildren in some way! Yes, I have eight grandchildren, and they all have their own little nuances and traits. Some have blonde hair, some are brunette and some are even redheads. They make me smile, their hugs are priceless and they fill my life with a mixture of worry, laughter and joy. They encapsulate and represent this theme for me and when I think of them, I get a sense of warmth, uplifting and pure joy! It felt so comforting and nurturing to hold them together all in my hand.

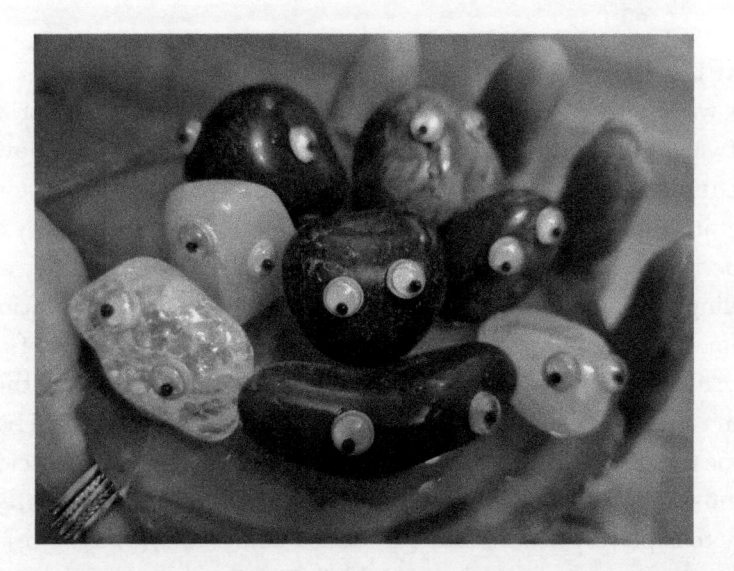

In our Creative Counsellors training, we invited five people from the audience to join us at the front of the room. We gave each person a piece of paper with a word on it and asked them to select a symbol to represent that word for them. Once they had selected their symbol, we invited them one by one to share their symbol and the word on their paper with the room. One by one, they shared their symbol, word and interpretation of the symbol, while the room sat in awe and silence. What they would come to learn is that they had all received the same word but had chosen very different symbols to interpret and represent this.

When I began my own transformational journey to integrate creativity into my counselling practice, I spent thousands on books, courses and products to help me to understand symbolism. I explored dream work, Jungian and Rogerian approaches, and anything else that offered some insight into how we process and make meaning of symbols, art, movement and creativity. What I learned was fascinating but what I was about to learn as I took this into my therapy room would be life changing for both my clients and myself. I learned that we can read as many books as we want and learn as many creative approaches and what they say about interpretation as we like, but the real magic comes when we work intuitively and realize that what matters most is what meaning, connections and understanding our clients express and experience on their creative adventures with us.

I have often been reminded of the power of interpretation in my work, and sometimes this can still surprise me. I have watched as people have chosen clouds to represent friendships, a black hole to represent excitement or a well to represent death: three things that I would never choose to represent those experiences. So, where does this all come from and what influences how we make meaning of our lives through creativity?

> **KEY POINT:** A client's choice of symbols, interventions and creative interpretation will be unique and individual to them.

OUR ROOTS INFLUENCE OUR REFLECTIONS

I grew up in various parts of Africa, and I am drawn to African beats, animals, bright colours, bold patterns, beaches and ocean life. I often work with these themes in a sand tray or draw on these experiences, shapes, colours and patterns to make sense of a situation, a feeling or an emotion.

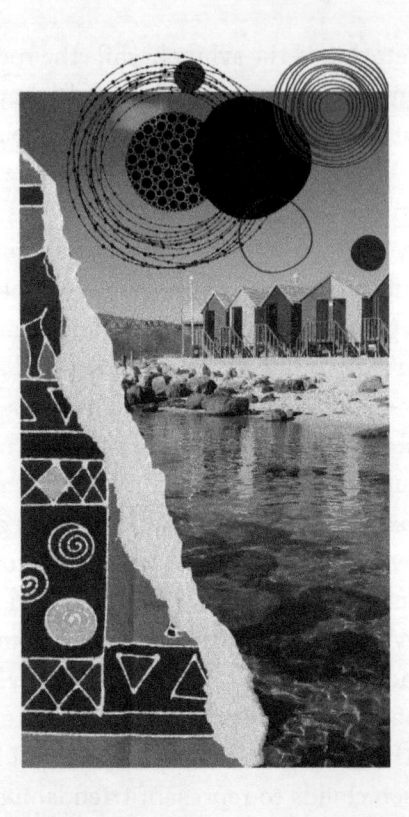

I remember sitting on the sofa at my boyfriend's house in Zimbabwe as a teenager, watching a movie with his parents. It was dark outside, and I was thinking about whether I should go home or stay until the end of the movie; I felt calm and totally relaxed. It was a really hot evening so the window was open, offering a gentle breeze throughout the room and I could hear the birds outside. Out of the blue, I heard a firm and loud command from across the room: 'Tanja, don't move, not even a muscle.' I looked up at my boyfriend's mother, who had raised her hand and locked her gaze on mine. Her husband had jumped up and run towards me. I froze in that moment and stopped breathing. In Zimbabwe at the time there were only a number of reasons that I could quickly make sense of in the moment for which I would be asked to freeze and I ran through all these scenarios in an instant. A gunman at the window, a snake at my feet, a spider or a scorpion. I felt every muscle in my body tighten, my vision went blurry and I could hear my heart beating in my head. In an instant, my boyfriend's father swept over my head with a towel, and I felt my boyfriend's hands pulling me away from the sofa as he scooped me up in his arms and carried me into the kitchen.

He then explained to me that I'd had a black scorpion next to me on the sofa by my ear. I was told that the scorpion had raised its belly and drawn back on its legs – a sure sign of attack. It had most likely been startled by me moving my head to yawn. I knew the damage and pain that black scorpions in Zimbabwe can cause: I had seen this for myself when a neighbour had been attacked. He had experienced respiratory problems, extreme pain for almost 36 hours and convulsions. I went into a form of shock, running through every scenario and what the outcomes could have been. What if I had moved too quickly? What if we hadn't seen this scorpion? What if they had frozen too and couldn't help me? What would have happened to me?

I struggled to sleep for many nights and still sometimes have nightmares about 'what may have been'. I became paranoid about anything and everything touching the floor, and this experience has stayed with me for life: it still influences the symbols that I work with and what meaning they have for me.

During a Creative Counselling training, I was invited to select a symbol that represents 'anxiety' for me, and I was immediately drawn to a scorpion. I struggled to pick this symbol up, and even though my rational brain knew that it was plastic, I still had a similar freeze response to being able to work with it in the moment. Choosing this symbol added an extra layer of 'anxiousness', which was great for the exercise and empowered me to feel and tell my story.

Each of us chose a totally unique symbol and theme to interpret and make meaning of our own anxiety, and although there were similar threads, like feeling something in our stomach or tensing our muscles, we all had our own meanings with their layers to convey.

In my experience, as clients begin to complete their creations, they will often look to me for the next steps. That look of 'What could this mean?'. Sometimes confused, sometimes excited and sometimes a little anxious about what they may be seeing, hearing, feeling or holding.

As we create space for understanding, processing and reflection to take place, we can work with our clients to explore in their own language, and there are various ways that we can do this through explorative questioning, nurturing prompts and check-ins.

🌀 **PRACTICE:** While keeping yourself safe and only working with what feels comfortable for you, I invite you to find five symbols around you that represent significant experiences, places, memories or people in your life. Take a moment to tune in to them. What do you feel in your body and where? How intense is this physical feeling? What are you most drawn to and why? What thoughts are you having? What emotions can you recognize? Do you remember feeling these emotions before? Are they the same or different in this context?

REFLECTING THROUGH MIND, BODY, FEELINGS AND INTUITION (MBFI REMINDER)

There are many different layers to reflection, and all of these are as important and valid as each other. For instance, we may feel a change or a shift in our body or we may notice new thoughts, memories, sounds or places pop into our thinking. We might experience a swoosh of new emotion, perhaps something that has been locked away for a long time, and this may feel uncomfortable, beautiful or confusing. These new realizations may feel subtle or they may feel gigantic, and each will bring its own gifts and shine a light on something that has perhaps been dormant and hidden away. We can help the process with our Mind, Body, Feelings and Intuition check-in! Remember MBFI?

- *In your mind* – Checking in with your thoughts. Are there any thoughts that are coming up for you now? Any people, memories, beliefs, places, for example?
- *In your body* – Checking in with your body. Take a moment to breathe and connect with what you have created. What are you experiencing in your body and where? Does it have a shape? A colour? Movement?
- *In your feelings* – Are you experiencing any emotions or feelings while you are creating or now that you are exploring this? What specific emotions? If you could rate your emotion out of ten what would it be? Can you describe this? Give it a name? A colour, a movement or anything else that feels important.
- *Intuition* – Checking inwards. What are you sensing, intuiting,

knowing in this moment? What feels important for you? What feels different?

> **KEY POINT:** Transformational reflection engages with the whole experience that a client is having: Mind, Body, Feelings and Intuition.

TUNING IN

As you continue to explore together, it can be helpful to support your client to tune in to various parts or aspects of their creation. This can bring even more awareness to what the client is experiencing.

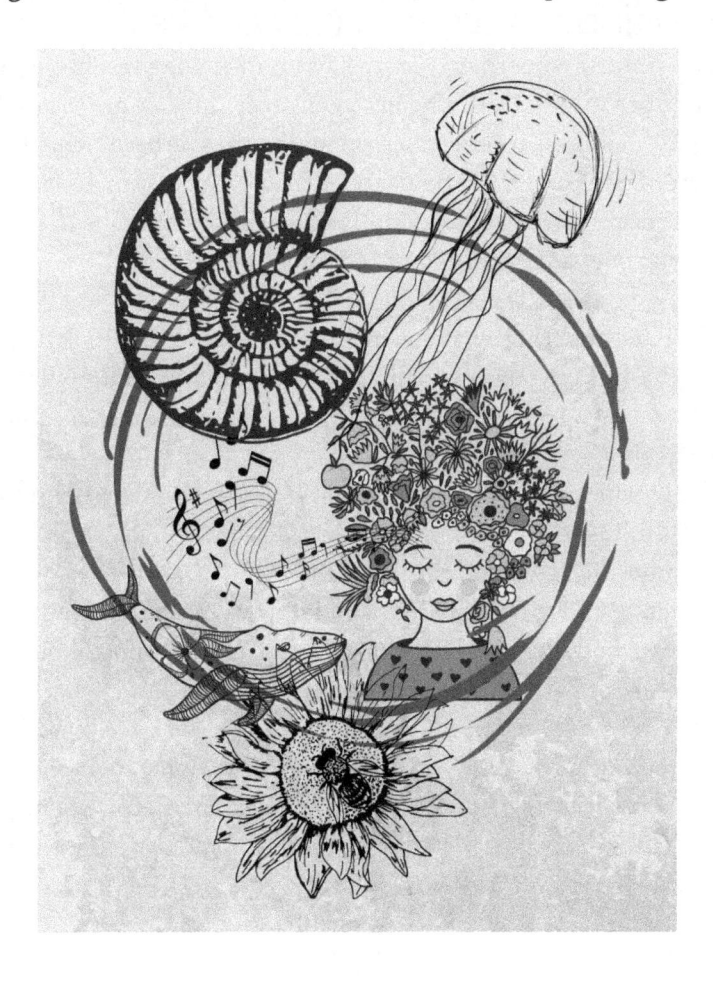

- 'I'm wondering what stands out for you the most in your painting?'
- 'If you could give your creation a name, what would it be?'
- 'Is there any specific part of your sand tray that you feel most connected to?'
- 'I'm wondering if you could talk me through your creation?'
- 'I'm noticing that some of the people in your drawing are much bigger than others, I'm wondering who they might be?'
- 'I noticed that as you created that pattern with the pen, you breathed much deeper than before. I'm wondering what may have been happening there for you?'

EXPLORING ANGLES AND PERSPECTIVES

When we create something, we are having an in-the-present-moment experience – mindfully tuning in to whatever story we are focused on telling. Sometimes, experiencing something that we have created from a different perspective can be an enlightening way to gain new insight, which is useful in Creative Counselling work. You may like to explore with open questioning prompts and nudges like these.

- 'I'm wondering what you might see if you were to look through the eyes of your symbol in the tray. From the position that they are in right now. What might this little oak tree be feeling, seeing, wondering?'
- 'I invite you to place your image on the table and to walk around it to see it from different angles. Has anything changed? Does anything feel different?'
- 'I'm wondering, now that you know what you know, whether you would like to add, change or adapt anything about your creation?'
- 'I'm wondering whether you would like to pick a new symbol to represent this new you that you are describing to me?'
- 'How does your collage look from a distance? How about from the back or the side? What is it like to stand and look over your collage vs how it feels to sit next to it?'

As we begin to facilitate a space to explore with our clients, they may begin to experience shifts in perspective, changes in their beliefs, new and challenging emotions, a deeper awareness and new understanding. It's important that we can hold and validate these experiences as they are happening in the moment while staying with the client's process.

VALIDATING AND HOLDING FEELINGS, EMOTIONS AND EXPERIENCES

I have experienced how my feelings, when they are not validated, can gain strength, take precedence and become overwhelming, and I have experienced how, when my feelings are validated, I can be supported to process and release my story in a much more healthy way.

As a survivor of sexual assault, I was terrified to return to school. I was scared of being judged and feeling different to everyone else. I was afraid of coming across my perpetrators and felt ashamed and scarred in some way. I remember being interviewed for hours by the police, and when I would try to talk about how I was feeling, I was told to 'stop talking about your feelings and share the facts'. I was totally shut down emotionally, so I took this into my life and numbed out any feeling and emotions for a long time. I learned very quickly that my feelings weren't important, so they gained strength and fuelled my beliefs about the world and my place in it.

We will all experience times in our lives when we feel invalidated because it feels as though our emotional experiences have been ignored, rejected or judged. These painful experiences or fear of these experiences can trigger the fight or flight response in the body, and this can create barriers to freely expressing our emotions on a day-to-day basis. This is especially true for clients who have experienced sexual violence, bullying, domestic violence, racial discrimination, traumatic school experiences and narcissistic relationships, to name a few. By the time clients have found their way to us, they are often scared of speaking their truth, because of their fear of judgement and rejection that they have experienced before. It takes vulnerability to share your pain with someone new and, for some, this emotional vulnerability can trigger the fight or flight response just as much as physical danger.

To add to this, we will also often have experiences of being supported by loved ones who disempower us without meaning to by offering advice or telling us what to do based on their own perspective. Although receiving support and a caring shoulder can feel good in the moment, it can often leave us feeling even more confused than before. Here are some of the well-intended but unhelpful statements people might make.

- 'Oh I'm sure that he didn't say it like that.'
- 'I don't think that the kids at school don't like you.'
- 'Awww don't feel low, feel happy – look at what you have in your life.'

I remember sitting on the sofa with a friend, angrily sobbing about an argument that I had experienced that morning with my partner. I remember how my friend had sprung into action, wrapping her arms around me and offering her words of support and encouragement, and telling me what she thought I wanted to hear. 'Oh don't feel like that, it's his fault not yours,' and, 'He shouldn't have said that, he has no right to feel ignored when you are the one doing all the hard work in this relationship.' The tricky outcome was an even more furious, newly empowered and ready-to-tango version of me – in the car and en route for round two with my partner, which didn't go so well!

I would later sit with a therapy student colleague and talk it out over lunch. What came from this experience was a whole new perspective on what had happened. We explored how I was really feeling and what impact this was having on me. We explored love languages and how I could communicate my needs to my partner. We explored what he might be trying to tell me from my own understanding. This colleague stayed with my feelings and emotions, validating all that was coming up for me in the moment, reminding me that all my feelings are important and significant. This created an opportunity for me to really tune in to my heart and share the hurt that I was feeling. What was really fuelling my fear? What would I like to say? How do I really feel about this? The outcome of this was a more balanced me, with a newfound perspective and empathy for what my partner might be experiencing, too. Armed with this new insight I went home to talk it out, and round three ended with us having a meaningful conversation around our own love languages and where these come from. This created the space for us to show up in our relationship fully, sharing all our feelings without any fear of being judged, rejected or ignored.

In this example, I shared the same presenting issue and was met with two different approaches. One approach that felt disempowering and invalidating in the long run and one in which I was empowered to make sense of my situation, my feelings were validated and I was able to make a more empowering choice in my relationship.

Clients will often come into the therapy room with a fear around 'not being creative', and as the space holders, it's important to see this as an integral part of the work we do while validating our clients' feelings and experiences throughout. For example, 'It's normal to feel anxious around being creative' and, 'I can sense that this is difficult for you to talk about.' However, creative approaches are incredible at validating our clients' feelings and emotions in the moment, as they offer a visual and embodied approach that encourages exploration, expression and connection. While our clients are creating, we can support this even more by actively validating through our body language, tone of voice and other prompts.

Sometimes, validation is simply a nod or a calming smile, and sometimes it's holding silence for a client without interrupting or offering a solution. Sometimes, validation is a nurturing compassion-based statement like, 'It's okay to have these feelings and all of your feelings are important.' Sometimes, validation may come in the form of reflecting back a statement that a client has shared, for example, '...and you share that you are feeling invisible and ignored'. All these validation approaches empower clients to begin to express and own their own feelings.

FIVE CREATIVE REFLECTION APPROACHES
Reflective Writing
Invite the client to take some time to write about what they have created or are experiencing. Encourage free flow and space to 'mind dump' what they are feeling and thinking on to paper. Suggest that they note any specific learnings, feelings, emotions and experiences that they have had.

Role Play

Sometimes, having a space to 'play things out' or experience things from a different perspective can be helpful. In role play, we can support clients to build on what they have created by adding an additional layer of interactivity.

EXAMPLE

Client: It's hard to explain how this bull comes across to the fairy when they are arguing.

Counsellor: I'm wondering if you could show me with your body language how the fairy experiences the bull when they are arguing?

Client: He crosses his arms and scowls, he becomes bigger in the room and his eyes lock on to the fairy's like this.

Counsellor: [Mirroring the client] So he comes across like this and how does the fairy experience this? Can you show me with your body language?

Client: The fairy wants to disappear into her wings, but they aren't big enough to keep her safe from feeling hurt and scared.

Conversational Writing

Invite the client to reflect on what they have created by writing a conversational dialogue between elements in their creation.

EXAMPLE

Counsellor: You share that you feel that the tree has something to say to the acorn. I am wondering what the tree would say to the acorn if they could speak? Would you like to take some time to write a conversation between the tree and the acorn?

Client: Little acorn, you are here. You are safe and you are important too.

Title Your Creation

'I am wondering what title or name you might give this creation?' This reflective question has always offered some powerful insight to support the work when clients are creating.

Photography

Invite the client to take photos of their creation on their phone and then explore this from a different angle. 'What can you see that you may not have been aware of before? What stands out for you? What happens if you change the colour of the image or zoom in?'

Whatever reflective approach you choose to support your clients to keep exploring the many layers of their creations, trust that they know where to go. Their unconscious mind will bridge the gap and they will take away what feels important and significant for them in the moment.

> **KEY POINT:** Trust that your client knows where to focus their reflections, what to process and how deep to work.

REFLECTIONS

- We all reflect in different ways, and a reflection can be as simple as taking a moment to pause or as challenging as asking a direct and challenging question. Take your clients' lead with what feels okay for them.
- Every client will interpret symbols differently and from their own unique perspective. Consider taking a moment to encourage your client to reflect on what each exercise, symbol or expression means for them.
- Trust that your client knows where to focus their reflections, what to process and how deep to work. Follow your instincts and nudge the client to explore reflections so that they take some time to process during each intervention. There is magic in these reflections!

Chapter 7

Endings and New Beginnings

In this chapter, we will explore the sixth element in my Create Circle Approach, which is how to facilitate and nurture endings as an important part of the process. We will explore planned and unplanned endings, along with some creative ideas for how to navigate this compassionately.

EXPLORING ENDINGS IN CREATIVE COUNSELLING

The waves crash into the shore, exploring jagged rocks and pearlescent crystal grains of sand. Then when they have gone as far as they want to go, they make their way back into the sea.

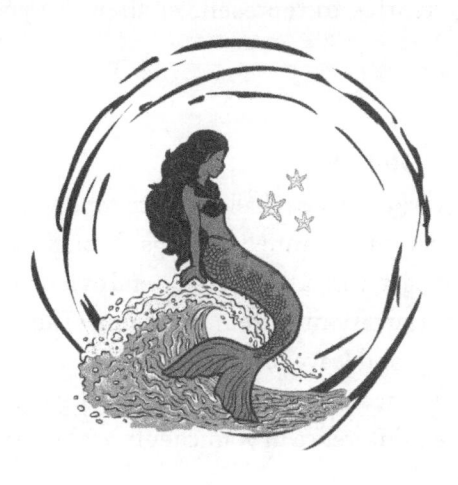

Just like the waves, many clients come crashing into the therapy room with a yearning to tip out their jagged rocks; an inner drive to explore their shoreline and find those pearly grains of wisdom that they have struggled to uncover alone.

Clients often come into the counselling room with a fear of endings, sensing them as a form of loss in some way. We are surrounded by examples of endings in everyday life, including a parent walking out on us, a bereavement, a loss of a sense of safety, being made redundant or a loss of wellbeing and health. However, endings, transitions, loss and change are a natural part of life, and we can mirror this empathically and within safe boundaries in the therapeutic relationship.

As counsellors, when we manage endings in a nurturing, compassionate and transparent way, we can walk alongside our clients to go as far as they want to go, before preparing to guide them gently back into the sea of life.

For many clients who have had negative experiences and may even fear endings, we can model a nurturing ending that offers a different perspective that empowers and prepares them over time to see endings as a natural part of the therapy process and not another form of loss.

Endings can also be impacted by the therapist's own experiences of endings, and it can be helpful to be aware of your own thoughts and feelings around this.

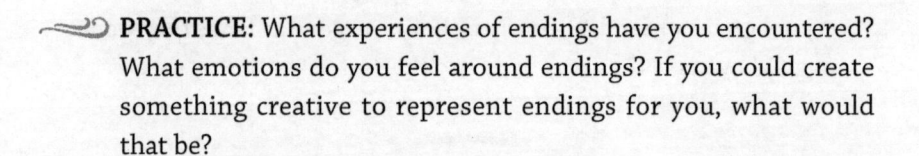

PRACTICE: What experiences of endings have you encountered? What emotions do you feel around endings? If you could create something creative to represent endings for you, what would that be?

PLANNED ENDINGS

Planned endings are often less challenging to cope with than unplanned endings. We experience planned endings throughout life, including retirement, moving in with a partner (the end of living independently), getting married (transitioning from being single) and watching a child spread their wings and leave for university.

We can experience something similar in the therapy room. You will often notice a difference in your clients as they approach the end of their therapy. They may start to miss appointments or reschedule often. They may start to use language that demonstrates growth and transformation. We can see examples of planned endings in agencies that offer time-limited sessions or as clients grow through counselling and come to a natural end. Planned endings empower clients to feel supported. They provide us with the opportunity to nurture clients all the way through the process.

UNPLANNED ENDINGS

Unplanned endings can be trickier to manage. They often leave open wounds for clients and can create a sense of unfinished business. Examples of unplanned endings include a counselling service closing down, a counsellor becoming unwell or the client leaving without any communication. For the purpose of this book, we are going to explore creative interventions to support planned endings.

Nature shares with us many examples of creative and natural endings that we can take inspiration from for counselling and therapy work. The sun rising and setting on each new day, storms marching in, calming, and passing and the seasons changing are all beautiful ways that the world shares with us that all endings have a beginning, and this is where we sow the seed for the endings process in counselling: *at the beginning*.

CONTRACTING AND GOAL SETTING

In Chapters 3 and 4, we explored contracting and goals setting. For the purpose of exploring endings, we will revisit some of the concepts that are most useful for us here.

The contracting process in the first session is crucial to setting the foundations for how we will work together, and part of this process includes preparing our clients for the end of therapy. We do this in a number of ways. We agree on when we will meet, where and for how long, setting the tone for beginnings and endings in each session. We set goals and negotiate shared boundaries, which includes preparing for a planned ending. We navigate our cancellations policy, facilitating our client's right to choose when to end their sessions, and we discuss how many sessions we will contract for and referrals if a client finds that they may need a different approach or counsellor. Without exploring the end, we have not really begun the therapy at all!

The BACP *Ethical Framework for the Counselling Professions* (2018) asks us to work with clients to agree and explore the number of sessions as part of the contracting process and to do our best to inform clients well in advance of approaching endings, while being sensitive to any expectations and concerns when we are approaching the end of our work together. This framing ensures that clients can be autonomous within the relationship and that we fully support them along the journey. Working creatively in counselling also presents a unique set of challenges that we have to navigate with our clients to offer a safe and therapeutic relationship.

> **KEY POINT:** Endings in counselling start at the beginning.

CONFIDENTIALITY

Clients are often sharing their most vulnerable selves with us. They are sharing their stories, their pain, their experiences and their most hidden truths. When working creatively, we work in a deeper way, often experiencing a client's emotional map from a full sensory approach. We may see their perpetrator come to life in a piece of art. We might hear their deepest sadness as they beat a drum, and we may find ourselves holding their inner child safely within a nesting doll while they create a sandcastle home for her to begin to heal in.

We are constantly helping to bridge the gap between the unconscious and the conscious, and although words resonate deeply, they come and go in the space, leaving an invisible mark when clients leave the room. When working creatively, we are almost always ending sessions with a confidentiality dilemma. As counsellors, we are all bound to offer confidentiality to our clients to ensure that their information stays anonymous and to prevent any harm. This includes the way in which we send and store emails, our phone conversations and the way in which we keep our client logs, take notes and explore client work in supervision sessions. The more experience we gain, the more routine this becomes, and we all have our own unique way of addressing these challenges. As Creative Counsellors, we often face significant challenges in how we store client creations. It's one thing to consider how we store paperwork and notes but a whole different set of complications arise when we are asked to store work that a client has created during session. This could be large pieces of artwork or images, photos and symbols that they have worked with or brought with them.

So, how do we store a volcano that has been created from clay, topped with tiny symbols that represent each family member, and that is currently oozing with angry lava, when a client is still working on this and does not feel safe taking it home? Maybe their partner is one of those tiny symbols. Maybe their child is represented by the angry lava. Maybe the client does not yet fully trust themselves with their fiery volcano. Maybe a client has a need to be held emotionally while exploring their volcano and senses that they are not able to do this safely at home, away from sessions. There are many reasons why a client may be expressing their desire for us as counsellors to hold their creations for them, and this is an opportunity to deepen our therapeutic relationship, build on trust and explore the process of change and transformation together.

In our Creative Counsellors Community, a popular question that pops up time and time again is: 'Just how do we support clients to store their creations at the end of each session?'.

PHYSICAL SPACE AND ENVIRONMENT

As Creative Counsellors, we need to recognize the challenges and any limitations on what we can offer to our clients. It is especially important to begin by considering our physical space and environment. Some key questions to consider are given here.

- Can I store client work and, if so, how?
- Can I ensure confidentiality of stored client work?
- How long can I store this for?
- Is the creative intervention that I am suggesting appropriate for managing the ending of the exercise and the session?
- Have I discussed this openly with my client?

In my experience, working creatively means clients often gain new insight into how they think and feel about a problem they have because they witness the solution untangling itself through the creative intervention. Because of this, clients often develop a deep bond with what they have created, and we need to manage this sensitively, with empathy and compassion. Some clients may wish to rip up their drawings and put them through a shredder and others may wish to keep them safe and secure while they process their thoughts and emotions.

STORING CLIENT WORK

A great way to support clients while managing expectations is to provide a visual representation of how you might store their creations in between sessions should they want to leave them with you. If it's not possible to leave creations with you, it is important to discuss this during contracting.

As part of the contracting process, I guide clients around the room, exploring different ways of working and discussing ways that we may store client work. One of the options that I offer is a personalized A3 client folder for artwork, as well as a storage box for any items created that they may want to keep safe.

These boxes are plain brown A3-size containers. I have found that showing clients the boxes means they automatically work in a way that manages these boundaries. The last thing we want to do is facilitate an exercise for our clients that opens new wounds and unearths fears and emotions that cannot safely be managed and stored as the client is leaving the room. It is much safer to manage these expectations at the beginning of your work together.

> **KEY POINT:** Consider your creative space and manage client expectations with regard to storing client work during your contracting.

PLACING SYMBOLS

When working with symbols, consider that the elephant that your client is nurturing gently in their hand is not a *representation* of their lost loved one but, in this moment, *is* their loved one. Right now, in this space, the client has removed the barrier that separates the elephant from their loved one, and we can see this in how our clients work with the symbols with powerful emotion and dedication.

In our Creative Counsellors 'Working Creatively with Symbols' training, we role play a scenario in which a client is exploring their relationship with their parent. The client has been sharing their pain around how they experience anger from their parent and how they desperately want to be unconditionally loved and held. Their parent is represented in one hand as a sharp, rugged and murky crystal stone and in the other hand they present themselves as a small, clear and transparent stone. During the role play, the client places themselves on their parent's stone and they sit there for a moment while they are being held. Two stones together as one. A deep healing taking place.

As this role play comes to an end, we demonstrate two scenarios. In the first ending, the counsellor lets the client know that they have come to the end of their session together and reaches over and collects both symbols from their client's hands. At this point, you can feel that the audience becomes uncomfortable, and there is often a sense of shock at the abrupt nature of the ending. A sense of interrupting the healing and 'handling' of both the parent and the client. With no regard for the client's process, this can demonstrate how we can cause trauma and harm to clients if we are not aware of the power of managing endings in Creative Counselling. The second scenario offers a much more nurturing and compassionate approach in which the counsellor lets the client know that they are coming to an end. They warmly invite the client to think about how they would like to end the session. They ask what the client would like to do with their symbols. They support the client to place the symbols back wherever they like and, just as importantly, to place them in any way that they feel comfortable with. The client places the symbols back together and with their parent still cradling them safely. In this scenario, the client would most likely leave the session with a sense of safety and healing, and the transformation would likely continue between the sessions.

You can sense the tension in the room visibly easing as this scenario is powerfully played out with respect and empathy.

This example demonstrates some key areas to be mindful of when working with and ending sessions with symbols.

- Let your client know that your session is coming to an end with a gentle, 'We have a few minutes remaining.'
- Invite your client to express any unfinished work with a nudge for final messages or actions.
- Invite your client to complete the process by placing their symbols how and where they feel comfortable to do so.

PHOTOGRAPHING WORK

When we facilitate an ending in a session, clients are often unsure about what to do with their creative work. They may want to keep processing their journey and/or want a keepsake of what they have discovered about themselves. They may have created an intricate sand tray, bursting with symbols brought to life through role play and emotion. They may have spent an hour designing a heart from clay or they may have been working to place cards to represent a timeline of their journey through life. Inviting clients to photograph their work can be a nurturing way to end sessions while maintaining boundaries and offering compassion in the process.

In my experience, this can be very empowering for a client in many ways. Clients have often shared that by taking a photograph away with them they were able to:

- share a part of their counselling journey with loved ones who were able to support them more
- continue to explore their feelings in between sessions
- keep a journal about their experiences and learn new things along the way
- look back on their sessions and realize just how far they had come
- recognize new skills and strengths they uncovered that they hadn't realized they had

✦ learn to trust their own judgement and process when it came to boundaries and sharing parts of themselves with others.

Many counsellors ask permission to take photos of client work to store with their notes, and this can be a useful way to make sense of the client journey. I have opted not to do this, as I make very minimal notes and can add anything that is of importance in a few lines within my writing. As counsellors, we all find our own way of working that feels right for us, and as long as we can safely manage boundaries and confidentiality, that is good enough. It's important to gain your client's permission to take photos, as some clients like to know that what they created is not being kept anywhere. Sometimes, a true ending is releasing the creation – never to be seen again.

ON SAYING GOODBYE TO OUR CLIENTS AT THE END OF THERAPY

As I am working through sessions with clients, I am always aware that just as the wave leaves the shore to make its way back into the sea, there will come a time when we will end our work together. Creativity gifts us a variety of expressive ways in which we can support clients to have a safe, nurturing and empathic ending experience. We are going to explore some of these here.

> **KEY POINT:** Invite your client to lead on how they choose to end their work and what they choose to do with their creations.

A Tools Timeline Exercise

In this exercise, we invite the client to explore key take-aways from the whole counselling journey, and I start this process with my client during our contracting, if this feels right. As with all creativity in counselling, you will get a sense of when and if the timing is right.

I developed this exercise in 2015 as a way to help my autistic clients to keep track of the learning, skills and strengths that they uncovered during our sessions each week. I quickly realized that this was a beautifully grounding way to support all my clients to recognize just how far they have come, as well as empowering them with reminders of the resilience and resourcefulness that they have within them to overcome any new challenges that they may face along the way.

See the 'Tools Timeline' section of Chapter 4 for instructions on using the Tools Timeline.

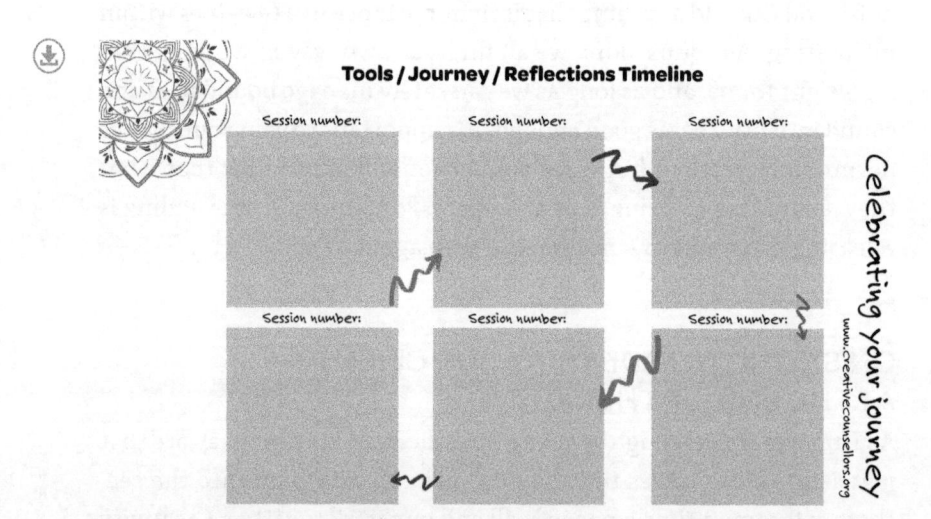

Tools / Journey / Reflections Timeline

Celebrating your journey
www.creativecounsellors.org

This worksheet is available to download from https://library.jkp.com/redeem using the voucher code: VLAJAFS

Exploring the Box

I spoke earlier in this chapter about how we can offer our clients a way to keep their creations safe in between sessions. As part of this, I shared how I offer clients a box to store their creations.

At the end of your time together, and if it feels right, exploring their box can offer the client extraordinary insight into how far they have come and all the incredible ways that they have grown over time. As with all exercises, follow your client's lead. Notice what items they bring out first and how they place them. Notice any changes in your client's body language and reflect on this as you navigate the box. What has changed? Helping clients to notice any changes can also facilitate a meaningful end.

Then and Now

When clients first arrive in the room, they often present quite differently to how they present when they leave the room. This can be in: how they see themselves, their hopes and their dreams for the future; how they handle difficulties and challenges; or how they approach their thoughts, their feelings and their perspective on a vast number of life's moments. This exercise is another inspiring way to support clients to recognize the change.

Invite your client to split a sheet of paper in two with a marker or pencil. (Notice how I did not say half: I have worked with clients who have intuitively split the page with a tiny proportion representing their pre-therapy self and a large proportion representing their post-therapy self or vice versa.) This is an important part of the process.

Invite your client to draw something on one side that represents who they were as a person on coming into therapy. Then invite them to draw something that represents who they are now on leaving therapy.

Notice how much time is spent on each area, the change in rhythm of movement across the page, and the care and nurture offered to each side. Explore anything that feels important in the client's process.

What changes does the client see in themselves? How do they refer to themselves today?

My Journey in the Sand

Sand offers us a creative way to bridge the gap between the conscious and unconscious mind. Clients can find it really empowering to recognize the parts of themselves that have changed. For this exercise, we invite the client to create a sand tray that represents their journey through counselling using symbols in the sand.

In this example sand tray, I chose a golden egg to represent my whole self and feeling rebirthed. I chose a diamond to represent opening up to life more, a golden crystal to represent growth and a harp to remind myself to be more playful in life.

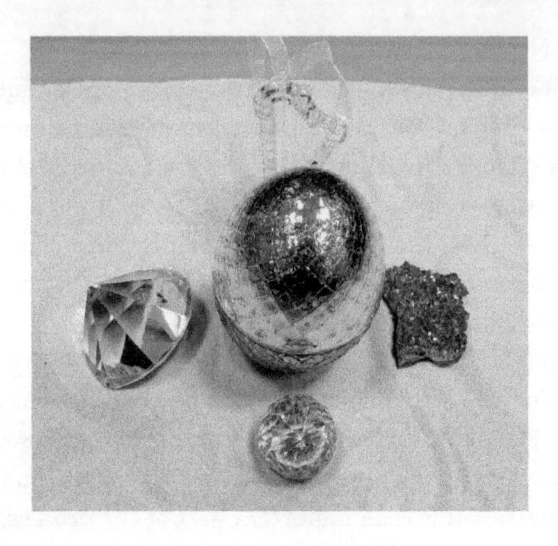

Energy Wheel – Things That Help Me to Stay Grounded and Well

In this exercise, we invite the client to explore all the ways that empower them to connect with feeling grounded and well. In this example, the creator shares that these things are exploring life curiously, having regular date nights, connecting with spirituality, exploring their wild side, calming colouring, recognizing that you don't always have to look on the bright side, taking daily mindful moments and creating daily rituals for a wellness boost.

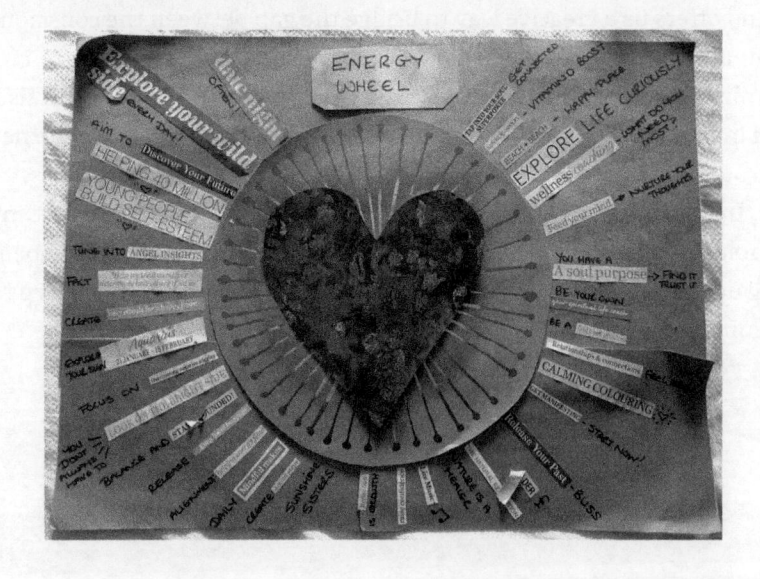

Working Creatively with Word Cards by Gaynor Rimmer

Gaynor Rimmer shares one of her favourite endings exercises with clients, Word Cards.

Clients begin counselling for a variety of reasons, and we work together towards an ending. As a counsellor, I feel it is also part of my job to explore a maintenance plan with them prior to ending our sessions. Initially, we go over all the skills and interventions they have learned and implemented during their therapeutic journey. They can be easy enough to remember in the therapeutic setting, but outside in the wider world with so many other distractions, it is much easier to forget the things that help us. Therefore, I create a set of cards personalized with words that the individual client identifies with. They are a visual representation and a reminder of all the strategies and interventions the client finds useful. This gives the client something to take away as both a reminder of their journey and a visual toolkit.

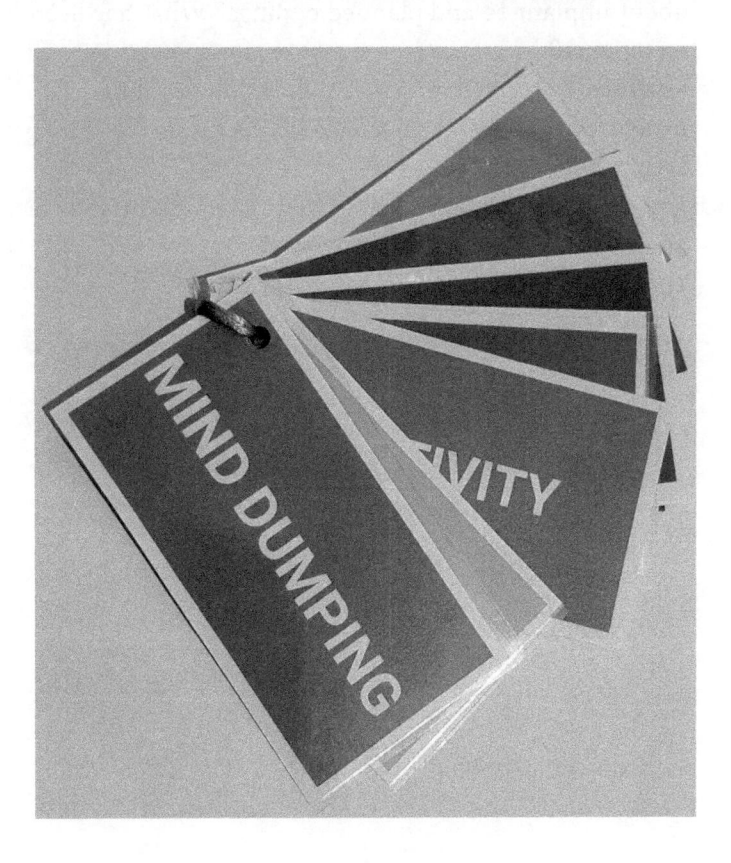

Now that we have explored why endings are a normal part of healthy life, we can see that if this stage of the process is tentatively nurtured and held, this can have a lasting and transformational impact on the client. Clients transition into counselling, transition during counselling and then transition out of the counselling room. Endings in counselling often signal a new beginning for clients, with clients exploring a newfound sense of self. Without managing endings appropriately, we can leave our clients feeling lost, rejected or confused. This is especially so for clients who have experienced trauma, struggled with attachment and/or have experienced significant loss.

REFLECTIONS

- Endings in counselling start at the beginning.
- Consider your own relationship with endings. How do you feel about unplanned and planned endings? What has been your experience?
- Consider your creative space and how you might manage client expectations about storing client work. Explore this during your contracting.
- Empower your client to make choices about how and when to choose to end their work and what they choose to do with their creations.

Chapter 8
Exploring the I in *CreatIvIty*

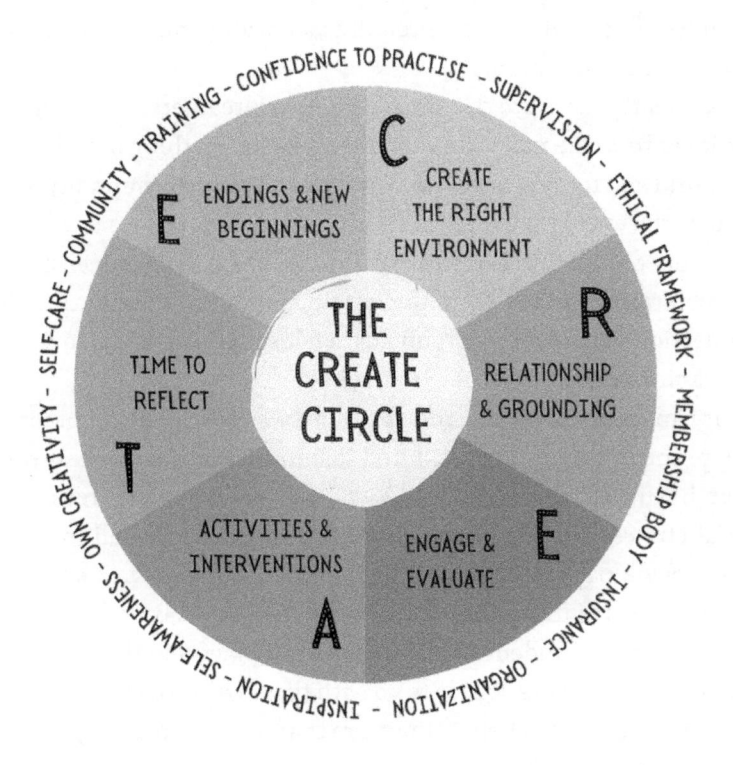

The Create Circle with surrounding elements:

Inner segments:
- **C** – CREATE THE RIGHT ENVIRONMENT
- **R** – RELATIONSHIP & GROUNDING
- **E** – ENGAGE & EVALUATE
- **A** – ACTIVITIES & INTERVENTIONS
- **T** – TIME TO REFLECT
- **E** – ENDINGS & NEW BEGINNINGS

Outer ring: TRAINING – CONFIDENCE TO PRACTISE – SUPERVISION – ETHICAL FRAMEWORK – MEMBERSHIP BODY – INSURANCE – ORGANIZATION – INSPIRATION – SELF-AWARENESS – OWN CREATIVITY – SELF-CARE – COMMUNITY

Throughout this book, we have been exploring the flow of the Create Circle, an ever-evolving concept that, although it first arrived in my thoughts around five years ago, brings more to my awareness for reflection each and every day. As part of this approach, it's also important to explore topics around our own passions, self-care, support and inspiration as Creative Counsellors. With this in mind, I created the outside circle as the boundary and the gatekeeper to provide stability and safety and bring a sense of self to the circle. Without the elements of the external circle, I believe that the internal circle cannot fully sustain its practice and thrive. It's the stuff that brings it all together, so we can facilitate spaces of transformation while thriving as *people before counsellors*. For the most part, this book has concentrated on client work, so this section is dedicated to you – to your wellness, to your success and to inspiring your own journey with creativity.

FINDING CREATIVE INSPIRATION

I believe that being creative requires a curious mind and a curious mind needs inspiration.

As creatives, we are the outside-the-box dreamers, the disruptors, the inventors, the magicians and the weavers, birthing our ideas into the world and forging a new path in the counselling community. For us to have the energy and the motivation to be creative, we have to find and connect with our own creative flow, and it can help to feel inspired.

Inspiration comes as an unconscious burst of creativity, a deep connection to something around us, a felt sense or a desire to connect with and recreate something that we see.

It can come in waves, and the more we look for it, the more we rewire the brain to notice it. I find inspiration in the smallest things from beautiful, ruined buildings, to the shadows that trees cast at certain times of day. I sketch everything for no reason at all and always have a blank-page notebook with me to doodle or write in if something catches my attention. This way of being creative has had a profound impact on my confidence to be curious and playful in the counselling room, and I feel more at ease to go with the flow and create in-the-moment exercises with clients. The more that natural creativity comes to us, the more inspiration we can experience and the less pressure we place on ourselves to be creative.

FOUR WAYS TO FIND CREATIVE INSPIRATION FOR *YOU*

Time to Do Nothing in Particular – to Just Be

I find that my busy brain struggles to be creative and is often judgemental and critical of what I create because there is no energetic flow. It's been a long road of recovery from being a 'doer' and I am still 'doing' my best to find my way to being – simply resting, noticing and being the observer. I have always struggled to rest and be still, and my colleague Gaynor once referred to me as 'being hardwired into the national grid'. I'm the person who gets bored while sitting on the beach and would rather be investigating the rock pools. Always a busy brain and so much to do! So, learning to be and do nothing in particular has been incredibly difficult. However, the most magical moments in my creativity have come from being this way. I am becoming more the observer every day, and this means lots of time for my brain to find inspiration in rest.

My favourite way to do this is to sit in my garden and simply watch what is happening around me. Taking it all in. The colours, the movement, the sound, the sensations, the taste in the air and anything else that I can connect with. Just observing. I began by challenging myself to a morning coffee in the garden with 10 minutes of observing a day, and this grew to 20 minutes, and now I can happily spend an hour 'being', which for me is a great achievement.

You might like to find a beautiful place in nature and watch the way that leaves journey down the river, you might like to visit an art gallery and sit with a painting to notice what you notice, or you might like to focus on a tree and observe how much life is happening all around this tree from its roots to its leaves.

Getting Lost in Colour

Have you ever noticed how many different shades of green there are in one tiny leaf? In Colour Therapy, we see that many of us are drawn to different shades of a colour and that they evoke different emotions, memories and states within us. I love to explore colour on canvas and paper, and in collage work, photography and observations. If I am looking for more relaxation in my life, I will often turn to light shades of green and mauve; when I am looking for energy and motivation, I will turn to yellows, oranges and pinks; when I am looking for healing, I work with teals, blues and purples. A beautiful way to bring more colour inspiration into your world is to collect images, photos and pictures that are abundant with a colour that you would like to explore or work with. Create a collage or place them around you and tune in to that colour. What do you notice and how do you feel? What tones are you most drawn to?

Sketching

I love to sketch patterns, shapes, shadows and simple designs. I particularly love sketching old ruins and buildings and found my happy place while travelling through the north coast of Scotland. The landscape there is dotted with abandoned wild wall structures, and I was drawn to the way that nature reclaims each individual quirky stone, with plants growing into them and around them. I will often take a photo of a building and then take some time to sketch and play on paper. This exercise is simply for enjoyment. On one of our Creative Counsellors retreats, I sketched a leaf as it made its way down the river, becoming stuck on every little jagged rock on its journey. There is so much metaphor to connect with here, and I take many life lessons from these very grounding inspirations.

Photography

On your next outdoor adventure, consider taking a camera and collecting images that inspire you. Maybe tree roots as they weave their way through the ground or interesting trees and their little hidey holes. Maybe you are drawn to open and bright landscapes or misty and moody pathways through the forest. You could combine this with colour matching and look for colours in nature that are similar to each other or are different tones. Simply collect images that you are drawn to for no particular reason.

DEEPENING YOUR SELF-AWARENESS

When we work creatively without self-judgement, we bring our whole selves fully into the room and all our senses are stimulated. We are seeing the symbol, holding the paint, smelling the clay, hearing the music, tasting the salty air from the shells in the tray, feeling the movement in the role play and sensing the story as it fills the room. I find that when we work creatively, there are many more moments of self-discovery that we have to manage in the session, and we have to stay aware and have a strong sense of self.

Exploring Boundaries

In creative work, I initially found that I was always working with a sense of being outside the box when it came to my core training. When I started working creatively, there wasn't any readily available information on social media or websites on how to do this safely and ethically. So, I had to become very good at thinking everything through and working things out for myself. As I learned, I shared with peers in our Facebook community and we would discuss things together.

Over the years, I have brought many of my own creative habits and interests into the therapy room, as well as certain challenges I experienced around boundaries. One of the most common dilemmas that I have experienced, and that we have been asked about many times on our training courses, is around the sharing of resources. I learned early on that to have a separation from client work, I needed to have separate resources from them. For example, I love to create sandalas in the sand for my own self-care and expression, arranging symbols and crystals unconsciously and reflecting on the messages that I would experience. I found that there is a sense of shared energy when we work with clients and mix our resources. I needed my own sand tray, resources, crystals and elements for my reflection – resources that I didn't associate with clients.

When I started, I also found that I would collect bits and pieces from around my home to work with as symbols in the counselling room, like old pieces of jewellery, stones and childhood toys. When I introduced them into the counselling space, I was surprised to find that I was secretively protective over the use and interpretation of these symbols, as they already had meaning for me. They quickly found their way out of the therapy room!

There was also a sense of connection to many of the materials, such as paints; I knew that clients were using the same paints that I had used to create my own art. So, I decided to separate the materials that I and the clients work with, and this brought me a sense of peace of calm. It reaffirmed the boundaries.

Working creatively also throws out other challenges when it comes to boundaries, like storing artwork and clay creations. Some clients request that I store items created in the session, and I have to balance this with considerations such as whether I have space available, the possibility that someone else may find this creation or the consequences of it breaking while it is in my care. I have reflected carefully on my boundaries around this, and I have included a discussion around it in my contracting so that, together, the client and I can come to an arrangement that suits both of us with regard to storing their work. It's also important to know about a client's situation, for example if they are in a challenging relationship for which they are in therapy, I would not work with a creative journal that they are invited to take home without exploring this together.

Time boundaries can be tricky when working creatively. What if you just haven't had the time to finish the painting? What might this be like for clients? Or what if you had to stop to manage a particularly emotional moment during your walk-and-talk session, meaning that you are running over your session time by 10 minutes and you have another client to see soon? I tend to plan for all these experiences and don't see more than four clients in a day so that I can give all of myself to my sessions. For me, this means a little extra cost to the clients that I work with.

When I first set my counselling rates and before I worked with creative interventions a lot, I did not have the creative resourcing overheads and did not need additional time to clean down and prepare a space for the next client. I also spent a lot less time reflecting on the whole process or doing exercises in the session. It is important for me to reflect this extra time in my rates.

For us to thrive as practitioners, it is important that we look at income boundaries, and it is crucial that we take them into consideration when we set our pricing structure. I charge more than I did before my creative days, and this means that I can source some great products and have journals, natural clay materials and a constantly updated selection of symbols readily available that I wouldn't otherwise be able to afford. I often buy new symbols based on a client's interest area or research materials to help explore their presenting issues. These all come at a cost, so this is reflected in the price. At first, I struggled with this dilemma, and I tried to offer everything at the rate that I charged before I facilitated creative sessions. This meant that I worked harder for less income. I learned quickly that this was not a clever exchange of energy, and I often could not afford the creative resources that I needed to fully support clients. I also often thought to myself, 'How come the GPs that I work with can afford to go on holiday and I can't?' Even though it was those very GPs who were coming to me for advice and guidance to support their clients! So, I changed my mindset around charging, and now I have a much fuller and better-thriving practice to which I can give my full self. I can afford to do nice things like travel and take a spa break to reground myself when needed. I also offer concessions when clients reach out, and I offer one free session per week to someone who is referred to me by the charities that I support. I offer charities free creative therapeutic video sessions and talks, so I am always giving back where I can and when time and energy allows.

PRACTICE: Take some paper and doodle yourself somewhere on the sheet. Create a bubble boundary around you that's big enough to place all the things within it that nurture and support you. On the outside of the bubble, doodle the things that come to mind that challenge your boundaries. Acknowledge the boundary bubble that you have created and update this regularly.

Exploring Grounding

Grounding is important for all therapists, and I found that working creatively required me to take my grounding practice to a whole new level. I would love to share some examples with you here.

BEFORE SESSIONS

I take some time to set an energetic intention that the client will experience everything that is right for them. I open windows and breathe fresh air into the room. I water my plants, play music and take time to set the tone for the space. I take a moment to imagine that my feet are centred, balanced and earthed, and that any and all energies that I experience are safe and grounded for me.

DURING SESSIONS

I will often shift my position if I feel that I need to reground. I might mention to my client, when it feels appropriate, that I'm sensing a need to check in if I feel that the energy in the room is chaotic, or I will sip some cold water and bring my attention back to my breath for a moment if I notice that I am holding my body in a tense way.

AFTER SESSIONS

I might open the windows again to invite a cleansing breeze into the room. I might take a short walk around the fields by my room and put my feet directly onto the earth. I might pat down my body or jump up and down on the spot. Sometimes, I may need to process some experiences and will free write around the session and then shred this. I may make a warm drink and sit outside or call a friend to ask what they have been watching on TV to reground my thinking into the here and now.

I believe that having a secure grounding practice is important for Creative Counsellors, as the work is often intense.

> **KEY POINT:** Working creatively can be just as emotive for us as it is for clients, and taking time to reflect on and grow our own self-awareness practice is crucial for working safely. Creative self-awareness can also be fun.

NURTURING YOUR OWN CREATIVITY

The more creative we are in our own life, the more confident we are to facilitate the space in Creative Counselling.

We get asked all the time: 'How do you build your own creativity for yourself so that you can help others in the counselling room?'. We have plenty of inspiration around this online in our Creative Counsellors Membership Hub, and I want to share some creative prompts that can help you to focus on your own creativity and inspire you to support your client work.

20 PROMPTS TO BOOST CREATIVITY FOR *YOU*

I invite you to have a range of resources to explore these prompts: permanent markers, paints, collage paper, newspapers, old magazines, pastels, glue and anything else that you are drawn to working with. It may help to have an art journal to create these in, as this could become an ongoing creative space for exploration. An art journal is a book big enough for your creations; I love using A4 size as it's big enough to work in and small enough to store away!

1. *Comforting Colours* – Find a photo that brings you feelings of comfort and joy. Recreate this in an abstract image in your journal. Find the colours that stand out for you in the image and add these as the background to your paper. Then add any other shapes or elements that you are drawn to and give this creation a title.
2. *My Power Animal* – Close your eyes and tune in to your body. What animal comes to mind for you when you think about your own personal power animal? This would be the animal that you evoke when you need a little extra empowering. Sketch, draw, paint or doodle your inner power animal. Does it have a name?
3. *Peace Garden* – Create a space at home for reflection. A peace garden that you can visit any time you need a little extra relaxation. What colours bring you peace? Paint some stones to add to the garden. Is there anything else that you would like to add?

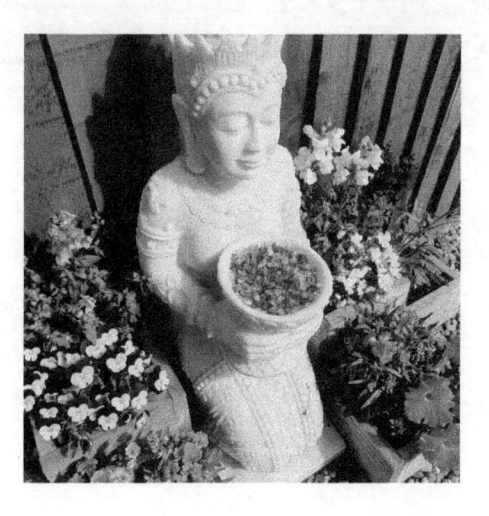

4. *Your Power Five* – In Africa, we have the power five: the lion, elephant, rhinoceros, leopard and Cape buffalo. Who are the power five in your life? The five people (or elements) that are there for you no matter what? The five that have your back and empower you! They give as much as they take, and they refill your self-care cup when you are with them.
5. *Melody* – Do you have a favourite song/sound/music? Play this and think about the following prompts. What colour comes to mind when you are listening to this? Add this to your creation. What memories come to mind? Add these. What people, places, feelings, images or anything else come to mind? Add these. Do you want to add any lyrics that stand out most for you?
6. *Collage* – Browse a magazine that you like (I love travel and holiday magazines!). Cut out any images, words and quotes that draw your attention. Create a collage in your journal and add layers like paint, collage paper, words, pastel, dried flowers or anything else that you feel inspired by. Does this creation have a title?
7. *My Place in Nature* – Take a photo of you in nature. Observe any feelings that you experience when you look at this image. Notice any thoughts that come to mind. Maybe give this a title.

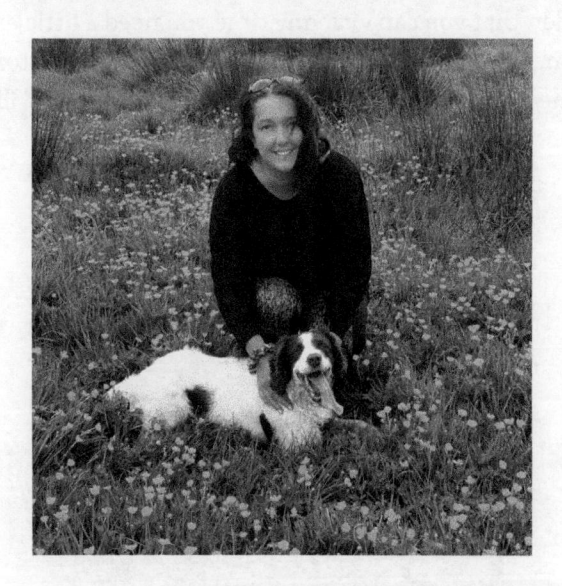

8. *Secret Garden* – Collect petals, leaves and other natural materials. Stick, paint, doodle, write, draw and create your own secret garden in your journal.
9. *Shooting Stars* – Create a night scene in your journal with colours that evoke a magical starry night for you. Then flick some lighter white, silver and yellow paint splashes on your pages to create a starry night sky. Is there anything else that you want to add?
10. *Create What You See* – Find somewhere that brings you a sense of being connected to your environment. Observe what you see, and draw, paint, sketch or doodle this. When I did this, I sat in my garden, looked across the field and was drawn to the trees and the buildings in the garden opposite.

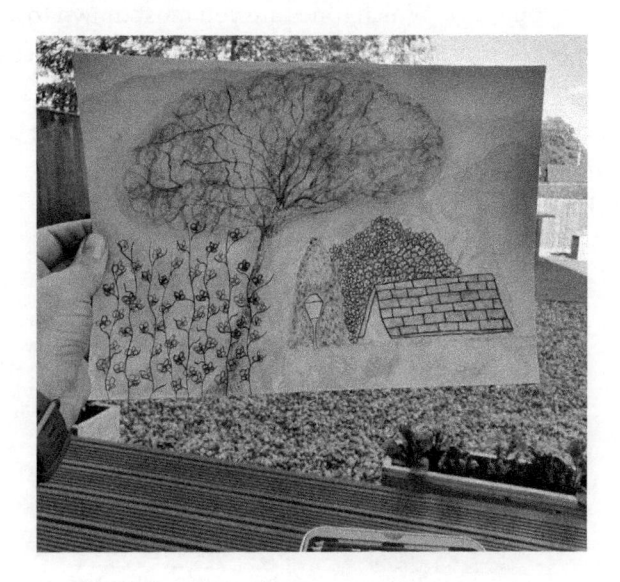

11. *Dream Doodles* – Connect with a dream that you have had and recreate the elements of the dream in your journal. What stands out most for you? Who was there? What colours, smells or other sensory information did you experience?
12. *Movie Magic* – What movie do you most connect with in life and why? For me, this has to be *Cool Runnings*. If you haven't seen this, it is a 1993 film about four Jamaican bobsleighers who dream of competing in the Winter Olympics, despite never

having seen snow. There is one moment in the film that I connect with most: when they arrive in Calgary to a frozen, white city after leaving a sunny, hot Jamaica. They are so cold that they end up in what looks like a hundred layers of clothing, and they are deeply out of their comfort zone. I connect with this feeling when I am being challenged to do something that tests my resilience. That sense of 'Yes, this isn't easy, and I can still choose to show up.' Dedicate a page to exploring a film that you are drawn to. What is it about the film that captivates you? What learnings do you take from the film? This is a great self-awareness and reflective exercise, too.

13. *Colour Mood Board* – Working with various colours, create your own colour mood board by layering broad strokes of colour across your page. Which tones are you most drawn to and why?
14. *Word Focus* – Think of a word that you would like to focus on and create something that represents this word. For this exercise, I focused on the word 'happy'. I added all the things to my life that bring me happiness and the colours that inspire happiness within me too.

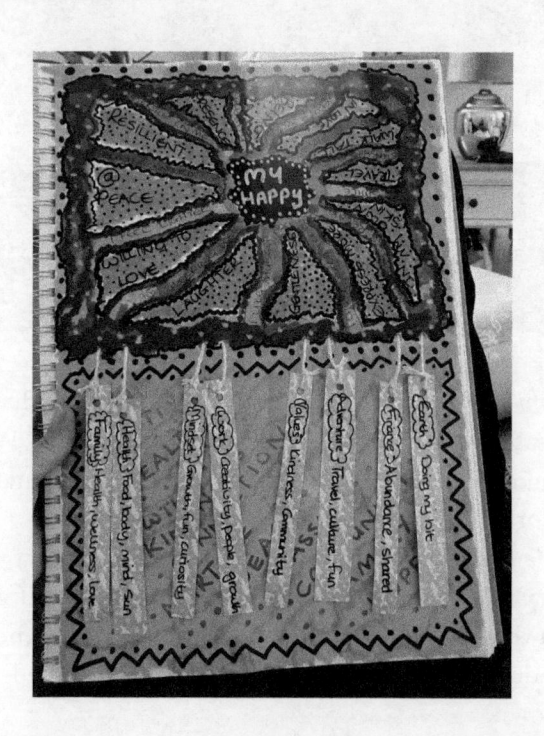

15. *I AM Mandala* – Create a mandala shape that you are drawn to. Add any colours, patterns and designs that feel important. Add an I AM statement to uplift and refresh you!

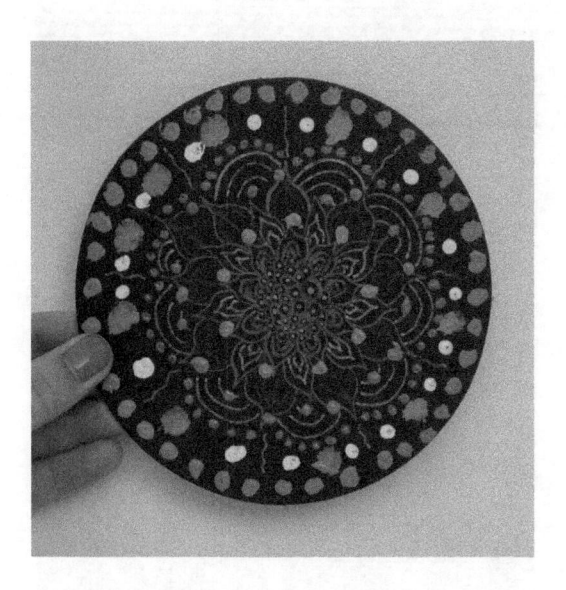

16. *My Sacred Space* – On the page, recreate a prayer or mantra that inspires you using images, colours that you connect with and words that feel healing to you.
17. *It's a Sweet Life* – Do you remember having favourite sweets as a child? Dedicate a whole page to exploring your sweet side. Add any images, words and flavours that you remember.
18. *Tune In* – Close your eyes and doodle any shapes, patterns, lines and movement on the page. Then open your eyes and observe. What do you see? What do you feel? Would you like to add anything to this?
19. *Your Name* – Dedicate a whole sheet to exploring your name. What does it mean? Where did it come from? If your name could be a colour, what would it be? If your name had a texture, what would this be?
20. *Create a Themed Sand Tray* – Think of a theme that you would like to explore. Pick symbols that help you to connect with this theme. Take your time to create a sand tray. Notice what you notice in your body. Notice any thoughts that come to you.

Notice any feelings that stand out for you. Does this sand tray have a title?

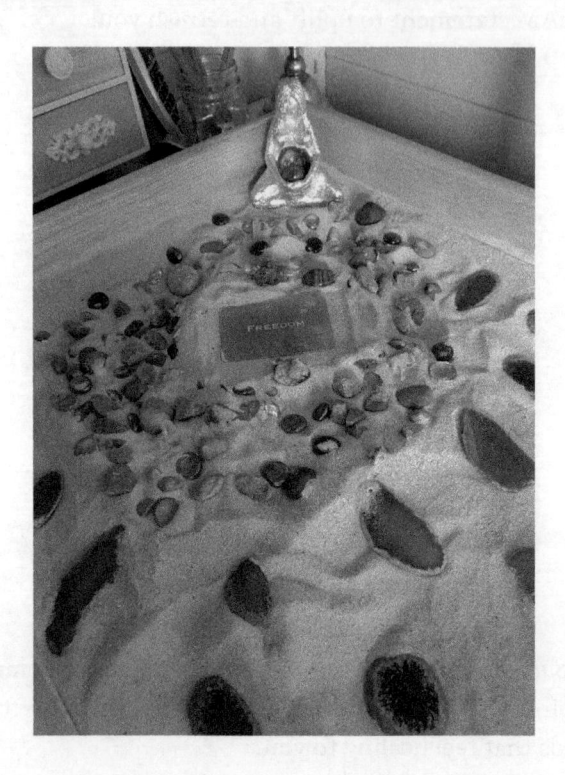

COUNSELLOR SELF-CARE

I have yet to meet a counsellor who did not choose this career because of challenges, trauma and adversity that they had experienced in their own life. We all have a story, and this often fuels and drives our motivation and is always working within us on an unconscious level. Because of this, I feel that counsellors are more prone to burnout, vicarious trauma and compassion or empathy fatigue.

Like many burnout stories, mine was a 'slow burner'. It crept up on me over time until one day I realized that I was spending more time crying into a cup of coffee than I was not crying. I cried for everyone. I cried for the whole world. I cried for my friend who was struggling with cancer. I cried for my clients who had spent an entire lifetime navigating the cold, dark seas of life in pain as a result of childhood sexual trauma. I cried for the many young, autistic clients

I was supporting who were feeling abandoned, judged and bullied by institutions that were supposed to be protecting them. Most of all, I cried for myself because I was too exhausted to do anything about it any more, and I could no longer take care of others if I couldn't even take care of myself.

Three months earlier, I had been in a car accident while driving home down a beautiful, sunny, country lane, with the music on and windows down. I had noticed that there was a car on my tail, swaying with me as we navigated the road. Looking forward, I had no idea that a truck was about to jump a stop sign and send me on a long journey of self-discovery. I didn't even see the truck that hit me, but I did feel it – every muscle in my body tightening and the most hideous sound of crashing as it drove me off the road and into oncoming traffic. I would find myself in A&E an hour later, strapped into a spinal board. I had broken the T8 bone in my spine and had a severe whiplash and injury to the right side of my cheek. I had to have three sessions of physiotherapy per week for a long time, and even though I could just about manage the pain, my biggest battle was managing my mindset.

I was overrun with guilt. The guilt of taking some time to heal and 'abandoning' my clients. They were on my mind every day. I struggled to sleep because of this, knowing that many of my clients were right in the middle of their work and telling myself the daily story that I was 'letting them down' somehow by not being there. Six weeks after my accident, and struggling with severe pain, I went back to work. I knew that I was still very ill and I still prioritized everyone else over myself. *What I didn't realize, was that by prioritizing everyone else's needs over my own, I was actually prioritizing no one's needs at all*, because I wasn't the same in the room. I was in pain and couldn't sit comfortably, so I was distracted and struggling to be present. I was filled with anxiety around driving my car, so by the time I would arrive at my practice, I was exhausted and well out of my window of tolerance. I wasn't sleeping well and so I was tired and foggy all the time, yet I still spun this story of how selfish I was to allow myself time to heal. So, the burnout crept in over three months, and finally I tried to get out of bed one day and realized that my body did not want to move. I knew in that moment what was happening, and I had no choice but to recognize how I was feeling and to start having some honest conversations with myself and my supervisor. We decided together that it was time to close the doors for a while; I still get a little emotional thinking about this. Handing over the keys to my beautiful and well-loved therapy space and saying goodbye to clients. Referring clients on to colleagues who could support and assist them and starting my real journey of recovery.

During this time, I went back into counselling to deal with my overwhelming feelings of loss, guilt and imposter syndrome. I was the founder and director of Creative Counsellors, a community that I was deeply proud of and inspired by, yet I was filled with anxiety and couldn't even get out of bed. I felt ashamed, alone and totally useless in that moment.

Just like the Wizard of Oz, I was showing up in my online work while hiding behind a curtain of self-doubt, but therapy began to help me to heal, and nine months after the accident, I was diagnosed with post traumatic fibromyalgia. Things began to make sense for me. I could begin to offer myself self-compassion again, and the exhaustion started to ease. Like Stella, I was getting my groove back!

I recognized that my body had been speaking to me all the time, warning me that burnout was coming, but I didn't honour its call! I struggled to tune in and to make sense of the messages, as I was too busy focusing on the external world and not the internal world.

Migraines: 'Tanja, your head's too busy worrying about others. It's okay, I can create an annoying banging feeling that will keep reminding you to rest.'
Fogginess: 'Tanja, you need to stop thinking about others and focus on yourself. It's okay, I got you, and I will create fog to keep your mind relaxed so you can heal.'
Tired legs: 'Tanja, you won't stop moving and doing and you are harming yourself. It's okay, I got you, and I will create dizzy legs so you have no choice but to stay in bed to nurture yourself.'

I finally started to listen to my body, and things began shifting quickly. Two months later, I would find myself on a plane headed to Facebook HQ in San Francisco after going through a three-month selection and interview process that led to me being recognized as one of 115 inspiring global community leaders who run impactful communities. I was on the ride of my life, meeting other incredible changemakers from across the world and learning more about how we could create a global space for counsellors to come together, to heal together and to thrive together.

A little while after that, I took to the stage with my best friend, Suzanne Alderson, to deliver a talk for UK Community Leaders at Facebook HQ in London titled 'Your Mental Health Struggle is Your Superpower', and I have been sharing this message ever since!

As counsellors, we gift so much of our time to others, and even when we 'clock off', our clients are often with us in our thoughts, sometimes sticking in our feelings and often being carried in our tensed muscles. Prioritizing self-care is as important for us as it is for our clients. I always remind myself that I want to show up in my life as my most vibrant, energized and healthy version, walking my talk and being a role model for self-care. I don't always show up this way, because I am human, I care and life throws us all challenges to overcome, but I do dedicate daily time to my own wellbeing and I now help other caregivers to do the same in our Heart Story® Creative Wellbeing and Mindfulness Programmes. Our Heart Story Model guides us through a six-part self-care practice that is proven to combat stress and vicarious trauma through mindful-based self-compassion skills. I have now trained 186 coaches worldwide to deliver this programme in their communities, and we have a thriving community of coaches to support this work. If you haven't already guessed, building community is one of my greatest passions in this life!

- *The H in Heart Story®* – Honouring your body's call and hearing what it has to say. Take time out each and every day to tune in to your body. What does it need in this moment? What is it holding on to? What does it need help to let go of? Complete this sentence: 'What my body needs most right now is…'.
- *The E in Heart Story®* – Exploring the whole experience. Take some time to tune in to observe or pay attention to your Mind, your Body, your Feelings and your Intuition. Even just 5 minutes per day can help. This is also a great self-reflection tool for checking in between client sessions.

- ✸ *The A in Heart Story®* – Acting with compassion. We often gift this to others and, in my experience of working with counsellors, we rarely offer this to ourselves. Self-compassion is like wrapping yourself in a warm, safe and secure blanket of friendship. It's treating yourself in the same way that you would treat someone else that you care for. It's holding yourself in the same way that you would hold a newborn puppy, with gentle care and respect. Offering yourself comforting self-talk like, 'Well, it's okay to feel exhausted, anyone would feel exhausted with the day that I had,' or maybe, 'I accept that I am struggling, anyone would be struggling in my shoes today.'
- ✸ *The R in Heart Story®* – Recognizing the truth! Checking in and taking time to catch any unwanted and unhelpful thoughts. Those moments of imposter syndrome and self-doubting behaviours. Reshaping those words and asking, 'Whose voice is this really?' and, 'Who does this belong to?'. Flipping those self-limiting phrases into more empowering self-talk that re-energizes and nurtures you.
- ✸ *The T in Heart Story®* – Taking action daily to make time for nurturing activities that refill your inner well. Nature walks, music, dance, art, baking, reading, writing or anything else that refreshes you.

Empowering Self-Talk Statements by Lin Sharpe

Lin Sharpe, a Metaphysical Coach, Meditation, Mindfulness and Spiritual Teacher, shares her love for working with empowering self-talk statements as a self-care practice.

As a teacher of metaphysics, spirituality, meditation and Mindfulness, I have learned that one of the most important self-care routines I can gift myself is starting my day in the 'right' way. For me, this is taking time first thing in the morning, before I get involved in the busyness and demands of everyday life. When we are constantly giving our time and energy to others, it is just as important to make sure we expend the energy remaining for ourselves in ways that support and uplift us.

There are some days when I need to be getting out early, or there is a time deadline on something so I am working early in the morning, and at these times, my day unfolds differently, with more bumps and challenges. On these days, I still try to ensure I give myself this precious time, even though it is later. I have proven time and again that this 'quiet' time in the morning can be the most important time of the day for me. It sets my day up with intention instead of allowing the day to drift, or charge, along. My mind is clearer and more focused. My body is calmer and more relaxed. There is a feeling of more empowerment and a knowingness that I can handle anything that unfolds in my day.

As I share this with you, I hope you may like to try this or something similar for yourself in the mornings, perhaps discovering how powerful and liberating it can be to make your own individualized statements and intentions. If you prefer, you could condense this into an abbreviated form.

Let's Begin

As we begin, you may like to find a position that is comfortable for you, where your mind and body can gently relax.

Begin by taking some deep breaths, really sighing out on the outbreath, giving your body permission to relax and let go. Now move your attention to your breath for a moment, breathing gently in and out, in and out, your breath settling into a gentle rhythm that is easy and comfortable. When you feel ready, begin this gentle inner dialogue:

> I now give my body permission to relax, my mind permission to be still and my feelings permission to come into more peace. Taking deep breaths, I allow myself to let go and come into this now moment as I begin my empowering statements and intentions.
>
> As I come into this day, I am setting a clear intention that this day unfolds with ease and grace, that I have all the skills and talents, the strengths, the courage and the resilience to face everything that life brings to me.
>
> Today, I keep reminding myself of the importance of being gentler with myself, of offering myself the same compassion as I offer others. Each day, I am willing to give myself more compassion. I am learning to treat myself as I would a dear friend.
>
> If I fall along the path of my life's journey, I gently pick myself up and give myself more gentleness, more understanding, more love. I acknowledge I cannot live on the earth without making mistakes. I learn from my mistakes and move forward with an open heart.

Every day, I am becoming more aware of how I think and speak about myself, whether internally or externally, and because I value myself more and more, I am choosing to speak to and think about myself with much kinder and more compassionate words.

I am giving myself permission to act towards myself in ways that support and uplift me on life's journey.

As I become more aware of what my own needs are, I am willing to take action to fulfil those needs as I remind myself that today I am choosing to look at myself with more gentleness, more understanding.

Each day, I honour myself as I am giving myself permission to take little pauses during the day, mini moments of Mindfulness. I choose what feels right in that moment, perhaps focusing on my feet connecting with the floor, or my breath as it moves through the body. I may listen to the sounds around me, or I may be aware of my body and what it is reflecting to me. I may choose to sit quietly, focusing inwardly for a few moments. Every day, I am willing to give myself these moments as a precious gift.

I am learning that my feelings are important and that as much as I can validate others' feelings, I validate my own feelings too. I am growing in my awareness of my own feelings and how I act upon them. Some of my feelings, I may choose to stay in for a while, yet others, I may consciously choose to replace with a different feeling. I can make new choices as to how I feel.

Today, I remind myself that I have the right to make new choices, and in this now moment, I am beginning to make choices that feel good to me. I am choosing to support myself with these choices, acknowledging that I have the courage to make changes or take action to manifest these new choices. If there are things I need to know to assist my choices, I take some moments to connect with my inner wisdom, my intuition, my GPS, which can guide me perfectly as I open and invite it to! I have the right to choose again and again.

Each day, I am beginning to open the door to more happiness in my life, in whatever way. I am choosing for happiness to reflect in my life. I am giving myself permission to experience more happiness.

Each day, I am choosing to experience more peace. I become more aware of the words I use, the thoughts I think and the emotions, energy in motion, that I emit. I remind myself that by choosing peace first, I am creating new neural pathways that will reflect in my life as greater peace. I have the right to take peaceful moments, knowing how powerful that simple choice for peace is! As I choose more peace, ultimately like a stone dropped in a pond, I am sending out ripples of peace to all life. I am choosing to be a peacemaker in this world, and I am grateful I have the opportunity to make this choice.

Every day, I remind myself to take a few moments to focus on gratitude and the people, places, things, perhaps experiences that I am grateful for. Focusing on gratitude opens my heart and raises my energy. When I am grateful, I attract more in my life.

In this now moment, I remind myself that the past is behind me and I cannot change it, I can let it go without judgement, freeing myself.

The future I am creating right now with my thoughts and feelings, the words I speak, the intentions I hold and the actions I take. As I am becoming more aware of all of this, I take myself gently by the hand, and I acknowledge that I can change how I think and feel, what actions I take as I make powerful choices, as I give myself much more gentleness, more kindness and compassion.

I remind myself to celebrate all my little achievements no matter how small, every time I have a new awareness of something, every time I take a few quiet moments, every time I pause and reflect, every kind word I speak or think towards myself or others, each time I make a positive choice or decision, all the little achievements each day and I am celebrating and congratulating myself, every forward step I take in life. I am worthy of my own self-love.

I am capable of choosing who I am to be and then acting on that, for I am much stronger, more courageous, more capable, more talented than I have allowed myself to believe and I love to remind myself of this as I journey through my life.

I believe in myself and all I am becoming.

I am at peace with myself for I am peace, I am peace, I am peace.

Taking a gentle, deep breath, bring your attention back into your environment and perhaps remain in this quiet place, allowing it to integrate at a deeper level.

I wish for you that every day ahead of you is a day where you just love to invite and expand your self-compassion, your self-acceptance your self-awareness, your happiness, your inner peace and all that you desire and require.

Nature Cups for Self-Care by Gaynor Rimmer

Gaynor Rimmer shares her Nurturing Nature Cups for Self-Care practice with us.

Creating nature cups is a relaxing and restorative creative exercise. Many people experience isolation and are cut off from the world outside. We all know the benefits of being in nature. The biophilia effect is our innate tendency to connect with other living things; nature cups are a great way to do this.

We can simply reuse old jars or teacups to create mini indoor gardens. We can create layers using pea gravel, soil, sand, decorative cork and crystal chips. The pea gravel is for drainage – the way we must let some things go in life. The soil is for nutrients, the sand is to provide a different aspect and the decorative elements are, well, to be just that – decorative and attractive to the eye. Finally, we can add small, easy-to-look-after plants and moss.

While I have been working from a confined office space during the pandemic, nature cups have helped reduce my stress levels and provided a more natural environment. They can be a hugely beneficial wellbeing practice.

For anyone struggling with isolation, creating a nature cup and adding shells, symbols or figures that represent our loved ones can be a nurturing way to help combat the feeling of being alone.

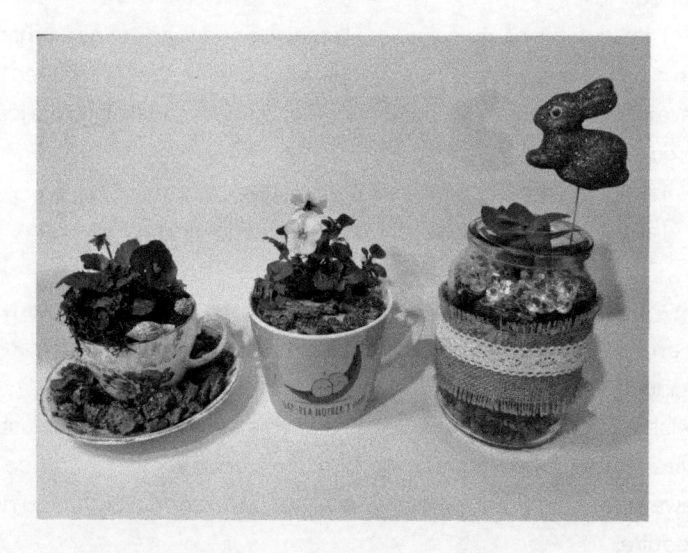

CREATIVE COUNSELLING COMMUNITY

I believe that we can achieve incredible things for the counselling world as a community, and we see the evidence of this every day. Claire Short, one of our community members, coined the term 'my counselling family' when she described the Creative Counsellors Community, and we take inspiration, connection and a sense of belonging from having a safe space to connect with each other.

- *Peer support* – This is about offering a space to share our most vulnerable selves and being honest, raw and real. A space to talk about how counselling impacts on us as therapists and how we can improve the world of creativity in counselling together. We plan retreats, gatherings, online virtual peer support groups and training in our community, and it's a relaxed, creative, nurturing and warm space to be where judgement, criticism and challenging behaviour are not tolerated!
- *Creative inspiration and training* – We host regular training in our communities to inspire and further develop skills around confidently integrating creativity into our counselling practice. We feature and spotlight our members who are going above and beyond to advocate for creativity in counselling.
- *Compassion* – We work from a place of compassion for self and others. Members share that it is difficult to find a space online that is free from criticism, argument and judgement, and we work hard to ensure that the community is a safe space for members to be able to ask any question without fear of being shamed or ridiculed. It is a nurturing space for reflection, connection and growth.

With these three pillars, we have come so far together. From that first night when I sat on my sofa and clicked 'create group' on Facebook, to launching our Creative Counsellors Big Ripple Project and organizing in-person creative skills shares across the UK, to hosting self-care retreats for counsellors in the beautiful mountains of Snowdonia and facilitating over 60 in-person meetups, all driven by what our community shares that they need most!

The community is the central focus of the work that we do, and I know that communities are changing the world. We will see more and more mental health communities coming together to create change, and this will have a positive impact on all of us.

When we stand together as a community, we create ripples that become waves!

TRAINING AND CONFIDENCE TO PRACTISE

PRACTICE: How confident do you feel right now to offer creative interventions in your counselling practice? Do you need support? Can you identify any areas to improve on?

I am a strong believer in experiencing any creative intervention for yourself before you try it with clients. This is for many reasons, including being aware of any triggers that might come up for you personally, recognizing your own process in the exercise, recognizing any blind spots around your skills and confidence to facilitate the intervention, and knowing what resources and clean-up materials you may need to facilitate the session appropriately.

It's important to recognize our own limitations and to seek training to empower us to offer the most inspiring space that we can for our clients. Every year, I create a wish list of training that I would like to attend. I often arrange for this training to be delivered at low cost to our Creative Counsellors Community or I might take some time away to refresh my skills.

We have been creating and delivering Creative Counselling CPD and training in person and online since 2018. Some of our most popular training workshop topics include:

- Creative Therapeutic Journaling
- Working Creatively in the Outdoors
- Working Creatively with Trauma
- Working Creatively with Nesting Dolls
- Working Creatively with Art Interventions
- Animal Assisted Therapies

* Working Creatively to Support Diversity in the Counselling Room.

We now have a CPCAB (Counselling and Psychotherapy Central Awarding Body) endorsed Creative Counselling pathway that guides counsellors through nine Creative Counselling CPD workshops over nine months, so participants can build confidence and come together to learn from each other.

There is also plenty of creative inspiration across social media platforms, like Pinterest and Instagram.

> **KEY POINT:** Take time to nurture your own creativity and then set some goals to seek out any creative training that will help to empower your practice as a Creative Counsellor.

CREATIVE SUPERVISION

I love how creativity can really support the whole supervision process. I have found that taking time to prepare for supervision creatively really helps me to make sense of what I am bringing to my session. Here are some of the techniques that I like to use.

* *Free writing* – Taking a moment to free write anything that comes up for me around my client work and process. I might write some poetry around how I am feeling, or I might revisit a dialogue in a particular session.
* *Sand tray* – I will often create a sand tray, picking out symbols to represent my client and symbols to represent me. Then I will take some time to observe what I see, how I feel about what I am noticing and particularly what stands out most for me to bring to supervision.
* *Word cloud* – I may create a series of words that represent my thoughts in that moment – my thoughts about my client or the process of counselling itself. This simple technique can really inspire your thinking around what to prioritize in supervision.

It's important to note how comfortable you are to bring your creative work to supervision. Does your supervisor respect your approach? Do they support you to explore creative interventions? You don't necessarily need a supervisor who has trained creatively, but in my experience, having an outside-the-box supervisor who facilitates a space where you can bring all of your true self as a Creative Counsellor is important.

Virtual Supervision

If you are working creatively online, you may need to check whether your supervisor is comfortable with supporting this different and often-challenging way of working. Many of our members have more than one supervisor for this reason, and they share that this really helps the process. It can also be very empowering to experience this supervision virtually yourself.

Walk-and-Talk Supervision

This year, we have trained hundreds of counsellors and supervisors to offer walk-and-talk therapy in their communities. We also have a dedicated Facebook community for members to come together to support each other with this creative practice. Walk-and-talk supervision presents its own challenges, and having a supervisor who walks and talks and feels confident to support your practice is crucial to safe practice. This is a different way of working, and peer support can really benefit your practice, too.

ETHICAL FRAMEWORK, MEMBERSHIP AND INSURANCE

As part of working safely I would nudge you to check your insurance when you are looking to work in the outdoors or in a way that may need some extra cover. In general, I find that insurance companies are great at assisting counsellors to work in wonderful, quirky and unique ways, and sometimes, clarification is key. There may be some limitations in the policy wording that need to be explored, and your most important point of contact is your insurance company.

Our Creative Counsellors Membership offers you weekly Creative Counselling CPD, discounted and priority tickets to any events, gatherings and retreats that we offer, a weekly peer-support and reflection group on Zoom and space to connect with other members to share in the process of creativity. We have a thriving community and membership who would love to meet with and support you!

BRINGING CREATIVE COUNSELLING TO YOUR ORGANIZATION

Do you work in an organization? Could you be an advocate for Creative Counselling in your workplace?

Over the years, I have gone out of my way to try to leave a creative thumbprint on any organization that I have worked with, supported or delivered training to so we can spread this incredible message around the power of creativity in counselling.

We now have a team of 15 Creative Counsellors Ambassadors, who are actively advocating for more creative approaches in counselling, and we would love to welcome your organization to the table for a conversation around how we can bring more creativity to your team.

Here are some other ways to advocate for Creative Counselling approaches in your organization.

- Start a monthly creativity circle or skills share. Invite other counsellors to attend and to bring a creative tool or intervention with them to share with the group.
- Contact us to deliver Creative Counselling training tailored to your needs.
- Create creativity corners in counselling rooms that include basic art supplies and ideas around getting started with creative approaches.
- Print and share creative resources in your staff rooms and share your ideas with your management team.

Exploring Creative Interventions within an Ethical Framework: What Our Research Says!

The following piece was written and researched for Creative Counsellors by Lisa Cromar, a Person-Centred Counsellor, Trainer and Researcher. She is a PhD student at the University of Chester, and is a published author, with a chapter in The Neurodiversity Reader (Pavilion Publishing).

I was excited to approach Lisa a few years ago to help me with a new research project, as I was struggling to find research in the field of Creative Counselling. There is plenty of research on Art Therapy and Creative Therapy, but my view is that Creative Counselling is its own beautiful approach that complements and respects the core models that we study, celebrate and value as counsellors (such as CBT, Psychodynamic, Person-Centred, Transactional Analysis, Integrative). This way of working combines our talking therapy approach with creative interventions, and the question that I get asked all the time is: is this ethical and how safe is it to work outside the box? At the time of writing this book, it is still quite a new and emerging area within counselling, and I wanted to find a way to map Creative Counselling to an ethical framework to act as a spark for future research and shared exploration.

I was full of gratitude when Lisa carried out an in-depth literature review, and I want to share a snippet of her findings here to open conversations around ethical practice for Creative Counselling.

Full article available at: www.creativecounsellors.org/blog/a-literature-review-exploring-how-effective-and-compatible-creative-interventions-are-when-combined-with-talking-therapy-creative-counselling.

Creative interventions (CIs) are combined with talking therapies on an ad-hoc basis. To ensure client safety, the research suggests an ethical framework is required to help allow for their deeper integration into counselling practice (Thomas 2017; Bastemur *et al.* 2016; Westergaard 2013). Andrew (2019) proposes an ethical framework which evolves from the BACP's *Ethical Framework for the Counselling Professions* (2018). This framework will be utilized to explore the ethical considerations highlighted in the research.

Justice

> The fair and impartial treatment of all clients and the provision of adequate services. (Andrew 2019, p.2)

The research suggests talking therapy is exclusionary to clients who struggle to verbalize their thoughts, feelings or experiences, whether due to the impact of trauma (Murray et al. 2017; Whisenhunt and Kress 2013; Sagan 2018; Kim 2010; Stevens and Spears 2009), developmental stage (adolescence) (Bastemur et al. 2016; Slyter 2012; Edgar-Bailey and Kress 2010) or challenges relating to neurodevelopmental conditions (Poquérusse et al. 2018; Winston, Mogrelia and Maher 2016; Hackett and Aafjes-van Doorn 2019). The integration of CIs into talking therapy appears to provide for a more adequate and inclusive therapeutic service.

Being Trustworthy

> Honouring the trust placed in the practitioner. Clients often feel nervous when they begin to do artwork, and we need to create a safe, non-judgmental space for them. (Andrew 2019, p.2)

Working with CIs could be unfamiliar territory for clients. They may experience negative emotions towards the process, fearing their creations may be judged; this need not be counterproductive. Instead, it could open up areas of exploration within a safe counselling relationship (Kwong, Ho and Huang 2019). Stepakoff's (2009) research with suicide survivors found that in sharing original material, the survivor does: 'not have to bear the pain alone… the therapist will bear…a portion of the pain' (p.111). Kim (2010) emphasizes the importance of conveying a non-judgemental space, making it clear that clients' visual and written expression would be accepted and respected, providing no 'pictorial interpretation or aesthetic judgment' (p.95).

Autonomy

> Respect for the client's self-governing. We do not force or shame the client. (Andrew 2019, p.2)

Kim (2010) elaborates on the importance of client choice in the CI used and for the counsellor to trust in their client's process. Edgar-Bailey and Kress (2010) agree; offering this choice can help restore a sense of control previously lost in the client's life. Research by Binkley (2013) suggests; 'counsellors should not push clients to discuss [their abuse] as re-traumatisation may occur, creative arts in session can give clients alternative means of exploring their stories in a safe manner' (p.312). Levy (2014) emphasizes the importance of counsellors learning to: 'listen carefully to [clients] and [to] let them teach [the counsellor] what they need and how to reach them' (p.26).

Beneficence

> Commitment to promoting the clients' well-being. We offer [CIs] because we genuinely believe this will benefit the client, e.g. in processing unconscious material. (Andrew 2019, p.2)

A counsellor may get a sense or be told by their client that talking therapy is too difficult or ineffective due to, for example, a need to suppress emotions. Research by Kwong, Ho and Huang (2019) using a mask-making activity with people living with HIV (PLHIV) found that a critical problem PLHIV face is the need to suppress and disguise their emotional status, due to the stigma surrounding the disease. The activity helped participants to: release, 'relax and stay attuned to their emotional status' (p.14). Further research by Edgar-Bailey and Kress (2010) with adolescents who have suffered the death of a parent found CIs useful to support them to identify and process conflicting feelings, such as love for the parent but anger at feeling abandoned by them. Leseho and Maxwell (2010) advocate for the use of dance to help the body and mind work together to form a connection that: 'would create a sense of safety for the body and mind to process information and emotions previously too difficult to face' (p.26).

Window of Tolerance

> The Window of Tolerance is a term coined by Dr Dan Siegel. It describes a 'zone' where a person's brain can function well, processing and integrating information and emotion without too much difficulty. (Andrew 2019, p.2)

Research suggests that greater awareness of a client's window of tolerance is imperative when working with trauma survivors (Kern and Perryman 2016; Ikonomopoulos *et al.* 2017; Murray *et al.* 2017; Paylo *et al.* 2014; Binkley 2013). Perryman, Blisard and Moss (2019) stress the need for counsellors to: 'maintain attunement and resonance, gauging clients' ability to stay within the window of tolerance, allowing them to express their feelings and to feel heard and understood' (pp.85–87). They argue that it is useful for a counsellor to have an understanding of neuroscience, enabling the monitoring of: 'hyperarousal, which includes feeling extremely zoned out and numb or feeling frozen in time. Ideally, the client remains focussed, alert and calm while recalling difficult memories' (p.89). Chong (2015) suggests working creatively has the: 'capacity to absorb and slow down... [hypoaroused] impulse emotions... [which helps] communication within the therapeutic relationship [to feel] less confrontational' (pp.121–123). Whisenhunt and Kress (2013) emphasize the importance of a strong therapeutic alliance and dedicating some time to helping clients develop the skills: 'to regulate the intensity of emotions that may emerge [they recommend] incorporating transitional periods into sessions [including] opportunities for clients to reorient and to become grounded to the present moment prior to ending the session' (p.132). Edgar-Bailey and Kress (2010) stress the importance of: 'developing emotion-regulation techniques, creating a strong, connected therapeutic bond and facilitating a reasonable measure of safety' (pp.172–173) when incorporating CIs into counselling practice.

Self-Respect

> Fostering the practitioner's self-knowledge, integrity and care for self. (Andrew 2019, p.2)

Perryman, Blisard and Moss (2019) explain that working with clients who have experienced trauma can feel overwhelming to the counsellor, CIs can provide a way for both the client and the counsellor to: 'remain within the window of tolerance for a longer period' (p.85). Kim (2010) agrees; when: 'facilitating a safe environment for the client...both the client and the [counsellor]... experience integration and transformation [aiding the] therapeutic growth of the [counsellor]' (p.98). Whisenhunt and Kress (2013) caution that CIs can be powerful tools that can: 'evoke intense emotions' (p.127), recommending that counsellors stay alert to any risk and be ready to support or intervene should the need arise: 'to hinder the unrestricted expression of anger and destruction when safety is compromised' (p.127).

Non-Maleficence

> A commitment to avoiding harm to the client. We don't offer [CIs] because we are bored, fancy experimenting or can't think what else to do. We work regularly through supervision. (Andrew 2019, p.2)

CIs can be very powerful and often result in emotions and issues being accessed more quickly than in traditional talking therapy due to defences being bypassed. Protecting clients from harm involves counsellors being trained to be prepared and ready to 'hold' their clients safely (Rosen and Atkins 2014; Edgar-Bailey and Kress 2010). Rosen and Atkins (2014) stress the importance of working within ethical guidelines, such as the BACP's *Ethical Framework for the Counselling Profession* (2018), to ensure the counsellor is working within their competence. Ensuring confidentiality extends to any artwork/creations produced by the client, and they engage in supervision to expand the counsellor's understanding of these interventions. Westergaard (2013) recommends: 'underpinning knowledge, understanding and experience... before diving into' (p.103) using creativity in counselling practice. Whisenhunt and Kress (2013) agree: 'adequate training and preparation are required [to] determine [which] intervention is appropriate for the client's unique needs' (p.132). The research demonstrates that training in the use of CIs is essential to ensure ethical practice and thus avoid harm to the client (Ginicola, Smith and Trzaska 2012; Bastemur *et al.* 2016; Kern and Perryman 2016).

Westergaard (2013) highlights that CIs are not: 'widely explored in counselling training' (p.103). Instead, there is a reliance on counsellors engaging in continuous personal development (CPD) to expand their knowledge. Rouse, Armstrong and McLeod (2015) add that there is a 'tension within primary training between addressing and enhancing the potential value of creativity, and the need to establish a sound base of counselling theory and practice' (p.177), see also Sagan (2018).

Extra Resources and Support

I hope that you were inspired to bring more creativity into your counselling room, and I would love to share some extra creative resources with you!

DOWNLOADS
If you visit https://library.jkp.com/redeem, you will find a series of short 15-minute workshops exploring some of the interventions from this book, as well as other downloadable resources that might help you on your journey. You can download these resources using the voucher code: VLAJAFS

CONTACT
I also invite you to share your experiences with me and send me any questions that you may have to tanja@tanjasharpe.com.

COMMUNITY
If, like me, you love being a part of a community, I would love to invite you to our Facebook community: www.facebook.com/groups/creativecounsellorsclub.

If you would like to find out more about the work that we are doing to advocate for more creativity in counselling, visit: www.creativecounsellors.org.

With love,

Tanja Sharpe

References

Andrew, P. (2019) *Integrating artwork into your counselling practice*. [Professional Development Day] 23/9/2019, Liverpool.
BACP (2018) *Ethical Framework for the Counselling Professions*. Accessed on 4/8/2021 at www.bacp.co.uk/media/3103/bacp-ethical-framework-for-the-counselling-professions-2018.pdf.
Bastemur, S., Dursun-Bilgin, M., Yildiz, Y. and Ucar, S. (2016) 'Alternative therapies: New approaches in counseling.' *Procedia – Social And Behavioral Sciences* 217, 1157–1166.
Binkley, E. (2013) 'Creative strategies for treating victims of domestic violence.' *Journal of Creativity in Mental Health* 8, 3, 305–313.
Chong, C. (2015). 'Why art psychotherapy? Through the lens of interpersonal neurobiology: The distinctive role of art psychotherapy intervention for clients with early relational trauma.' *International Journal Of Art Therapy, 20*, 3, 118–126. Accessed on 4/8/2021 at https://doi.org/10.1080/17454832.2015.1079727.
Cromar, L. (2021) *A Literature Review Exploring How Effective and Compatible Creative Interventions Are When combined with Talking Therapy*. Chester: Creative Counsellors. Accessed on 4/8/2021 at https://creativecounsellors.org/blog/a-literature-review-exploring-how-effective-and-compatible-creative-interventions-are-when-combined-with-talking-therapy-creative-counselling.
Department of Health and Social Care (2021) *£79 Million to Boost Mental Health Support for Children and Young People*. Accessed on 4/8/2021 at www.gov.uk/government/news/79-million-to-boost-mental-health-support-for-children-and-young-people.
Edgar-Bailey, M. and Kress, V. (2010) 'Resolving child and adolescent traumatic grief: Creative techniques and interventions.' *Journal of Creativity in Mental Health* 5, 2, 158–176.
Gawain, S. (2016) *Creative Visualization: Use the Power of Your Imagination to Create What You Want in Life*. Novato, CA: New World Library.
Ginicola, M., Smith, C. and Trzaska, J. (2012) 'Counseling through images: Using photography to guide the counseling process and achieve treatment goals.' *Journal of Creativity in Mental Health* 7, 4, 310–329.
Hackett, S. and Aafjes-van Doorn, K. (2019) 'Psychodynamic art psychotherapy for the treatment of aggression in an individual with antisocial personality disorder

in a secure forensic hospital: A single-case design study.' *American Psychological Association* 56, 2, 297–308.

Ikonomopoulos, J., Cavazos-Vela, J., Vela, P., Sanchez, M., Schmidt, C. and Catchings, C. (2017) 'Evaluating the effects of creative journal arts therapy for survivors of domestic violence.' *Journal of Creativity in Mental Health* 12, 4, 496–512.

Kern, E. and Perryman, K. (2016) 'Leaving it in the sand: Creatively processing military combat trauma as a means for reducing risk of interpersonal violence.' *Journal of Creativity in Mental Health* 11, 3–4, 446–457.

Kim, S. (2010) 'A story of a healing relationship: The person-centered approach in expressive arts therapy.' *Journal of Creativity in Mental Health* 5, 1, 93–98.

Kwong, M., Ho, R. and Huang, Y. (2019) 'A creative pathway to a meaningful life: An existential expressive arts group therapy for people living with HIV in Hong Kong.' *The Arts In Psychotherapy* 63, 9–17.

Leseho, J. and Maxwell, L. (2010) 'Coming alive: Creative movement as a personal coping strategy on the path to healing and growth.' *British Journal of Guidance and Counselling* 38, 1, 17–30.

Levy, F. (2014) 'Integrating the arts in psychotherapy: Opening the doors of shared creativity.' *American Journal of Dance Therapy* 36, 1, 6–27.

Murray, C., Moore Spencer, K., Stickl, J. and Crowe, A. (2017) 'See the Triumph Healing Arts Workshops for survivors of intimate partner violence and sexual assault.' *Journal of Creativity in Mental Health* 12, 2, 192–202.

Office for National Statistics (2021) *Coronavirus and Depression in Adults, Great Britain: January to March 2021*. Accessed on 4/8/2021 at www.ons.gov.uk/peoplepopulationandcommunity/wellbeing/articles/coronavirusanddepressioninadultsgreatbritain/januarytomarch2021.

Paylo, M., Darby, A., Kinch, S. and Kress, V. (2014) 'Creative rituals for use with traumatised adolescents.' *Journal of Creativity in Mental Health* 9, 1, 111–121.

Perryman, K., Blisard, P. and Moss, R. (2019) 'Using creative arts in trauma therapy: The neuroscience of healing.' *Journal of Mental Health Counseling* 41, 1, 80–94.

Poquérusse, J., Pastore, L., Dellantonio, S. and Esposito, G. (2018) 'Alexithymia and autism spectrum disorder: A complex relationship.' *Frontiers in Psychology* 9, 1–10.

Rosen, C. and Atkins, S. (2014) 'Am I doing expressive arts therapy or creativity in counseling?' *Journal of Creativity in Mental Health* 9, 2, 292–303.

Rouse, A., Armstrong, J. and McLeod, J. (2015) 'Enabling connections: Counsellor creativity and therapeutic practice.' *Counselling And Psychotherapy Research* 15, 3, 171–179.

Sagan, O. (2018) 'Art-making and its interface with dissociative identity disorder: No words that didn't fit.' *Journal of Creativity in Mental Health* 14, 1, 23–36.

Slyter, M. (2012) 'Creative counseling interventions for grieving adolescents.' *Journal of Creativity in Mental Health* 7, 1, 17–34.

Stepakoff, S. (2009) 'From destruction to creation, from silence to speech: Poetry therapy principles and practices for working with suicide grief.' *The Arts in Psychotherapy* 36, 2, 105–113.

Stevens, R. and Spears, E. (2009) 'Incorporating photography as a therapeutic tool in counseling.' *Journal of Creativity in Mental Health* 4, 1, 3–16.

Thomas, V. (2017) 'Towards a deeper integration of creative methods in counselling: Some thoughts about frameworks for practice.' *British Journal of Guidance and Counselling* 48, 1, 21–29.

Treanor, A. (2017) *The Extent to Which Relational Depth Can Be Reached in Online Therapy and the Factors That Facilitate and Inhibit That Experience: A Mixed Methods Study.* University of Roehampton, London. Accessed on 4/8/2021 at https://pure.roehampton.ac.uk/ws/portalfiles/portal/816047/Aisling_Treanor_Thesis.pdf.

Westergaard, J. (2013) 'Counselling young people: Counsellors' perspectives on "what works" – An exploratory study.' *Counselling And Psychotherapy Research 13*, 2, 98–105.

Whisenhunt, J. and Kress, V. (2013) 'The use of visual arts activities in counseling clients who engage in nonsuicidal self-injury.' *Journal of Creativity in Mental Health 8*, 2, 120–135.

Winston, C., Mogrelia, N. and Maher, H. (2016) 'The therapeutic value of asemic writing: A qualitative exploration.' *Journal of Creativity in Mental Health 11*, 2, 142–156.

Index

Aafjes-van Doorn, K. 203
Alderson, Suzanne 11–14, 25–6
Andrew, P. 202, 204, 205, 206
Armstrong, J. 206
art
    creative doodling 103
    drawing 84–5
    free-flow doodling 104–5
assessment *see* goal setting
Atkins, S. 206
Autonomous Sensory Meridian Response (ASMR) 94
autonomy of client 203–4

BACP 164, 202, 206
Bastemur, S. 202, 203, 206
being (not doing) 177
beneficence 204
Bennett, Masha 38, 94
Binkley, E. 203, 204
Blisard, P. 204
body language (during online counselling) 42
Bound, Mel 26
boundaries
    between personal and professional life 74–5
    during online counselling 44
    exploring 179–81
breathing exercises 65–7
bridge symbols 34
broken pieces (celebrating) 121
burnout 73–5, 189–90

cards 34
Cast Off Crafts 37
challenge board 107
characters 139–41
charging 180–1
check in, creative process, check out framework 70–1
check-in moments 58–60, 71–2
Chong, C. 205
clay 118–21
clay bowls 118–19
collage
    during assessment 83
    in online counselling 47
    for visual journaling 113
collage stones 128
Colour Bubble Breathing 66–7
colour (coding resources by) 39
Colour Therapy 83, 177–8
comic/cartoon symbols 33
community support 197–8
concessions (offering) 181
confidentiality 44, 164–5
contracting process 57–8, 164–5
conversational puppets 124–6
conversational writing 158
Cornthwaite, Dave 26
counselling models (integration with other) 17, 24, 56, 94
craft materials 35
Cramp, Cara 119–21
Create Circle Approach (introduction to) 21–2

Creative Counselling
   core principles of 23
   evolving nature of 20
   overview 17–20
creative doodling 103
creative pet intervention 109–10
creative visualization 132–7
creativity
   always present 25
   fears around lack of 24, 157
   nurturing your own 182–8
   turning away from 24–5
Cromar, Lisa 18, 202–6
culturally diverse resources 35–6

Dana, Deb 59–60
dance metaphor 21
Department of Health and
   Social Care 27
digital therapy resources 40
diversity 35–6
dolls *see* nesting dolls; matryoshka dolls
doodle stones 127–8
doodling 84–5, 103–5
drawing 84–5
drumming 95
Dunning, Tracy 126–7

Edgar-Bailey, M. 203, 204, 205, 206
embodiment 101–2
emotion cards 34
emotion stones 128
emotional expression 18–19
empowering self-talk statements 192–5
Empty Chair Cards 143–6
end of life symbols 33
endings
   exploring contents of box 170
   overview 161–2
   photographing work 168
   planned 162–3
   saying goodbye 169–75
   symbols at end of session 167–8
   then and now exercise 171
   unplanned 163
energetic intention 181
energy wheel 172
environment
   importance of 29–30
   see also indoor therapy rooms;
      nature interventions
ethical framework 202–6
explaining approach to clients 56

Facebook Community
   Leadership Program 25
fairy-tale symbols 33
fence symbols 34
fight or flight response 155
films 185–6
forest bathing 47–8
'40 Ways to Work Creatively
   Online' programme 41
free sessions 181
free-flow doodling 104–5
from-here-to-there exercise 85–6

garden
   indoor 196
   positive thoughts 52–3
Gawain, S. 132
getting lost in colour exercise 177–8
Ginicola, M. 206
goal setting
   doodling/drawing 84–5
   form-based 79–80
   from-here-to-there exercise 85–6
   hopes-and-dreams board 82–4
   my life circle exercise 80
   My World Creative Assessment
      tool 88–90
   nature metaphors 85
   number-range assessments 81–2
   sand-tray families/relationships 82
   trigger evaluation 84
grounding
   breathing exercises 65–7
   energy wheel 172
   grounding map 62–3, 76
   Mind, Body, Feelings and Intuition
      (MBFI) Cycle 68–9, 152–3
   overview 61–2
   sand-tray work 67–8
   for therapist 72–6, 181–2
   using sound 94–5
   using stones 130
   visualizations 64–5
   words 63–4

INDEX

Hackett, S. 203
Heart Story Model 191–2
Ho, R. 203, 204
hopes-and-dreams board 82–4
Huang, Y. 203, 204
humming 95
hyperarousal 205

I AM mandala 187
I AM poem 93–4
Ikonomopoulos, J. 204
images 34, 40
in and out of therapy 26
indoor gardens 196
indoor therapy rooms
    lighting 31–2
    overview 31
    sourcing resources for 32–5
    storage 37–9, 166, 180
    views from 32
    windows 32
inspiration (finding)
    getting lost in colour 177–8
    learning to be 177
    overview 176
    photography 178
    sketching 178
insurance 45, 200–1
integration with other approaches 17, 24, 56, 94
interpretation 149
intuition 71–2, 149
invalidation 155–7

journaling 110–14
joy (working with) 148–9
justice (in ethical framework) 202–3

Kern, E. 204, 206
Kim, S. 203, 205
Kress, V. 203, 204, 205, 206
Kwong, M. 203, 204

laminated photos 40
lamps 31–2
legal issues 45
Leseho, J. 204
Levy, F. 204
lighting 31–2

lyrics 92

McLeod, J. 206
Maher, H. 203
maintenance plan 173
mandalas 115–17
marketing 55–7
materials 33–5
matryoshka dolls 137–9
Maxwell, L. 204
memory boards 105–9
mental health issues (statistics) 27
metaphors
    clay work and 119–21
    nature 85
Mind, Body, Feelings and Intuition (MBFI) Cycle 68–9, 152–3
mindful poetry 98–9
mindfulness (during online counselling) 46
mobile counselling (carrying resources for) 40
Mogrelia, N. 203
morning routine 193–5
mosaics 121–3
Moss, R. 204, 205
Murray, C. 203, 204
musical instruments 97
my journey in the sand exercise 171–2
my life circle exercise 80
My World Creative Assessment tool 88–90

natural light 32
natural symbols 34
nature cups 196
nature interventions
    forest bathing 47–8
    ideas for 51–3
    indoor gardens 196
    nature as a co-therapist 50–1
    transient art 52
    wild play sessions 48–9
nature metaphors 85
nature's gift visualization 133–7
nervous system 94
nesting dolls 137–9
neurodiversity (lighting and) 31–2
non-maleficence 206

'not creative' fears 24, 157
number of sessions 164
number-range assessments 81–2

Office for National Statistics 27
O'Kane, Tara 129–30
Omijeh, Kemi 88–90
online counselling
　art 46
　body language 42
　boundaries 44
　collage 47
　confidentiality/privacy 44
　downloadable resources 47
　legal issues 45
　not for everyone 43
　overview 41–2
　role play 46
　set-up for 45
　supervision of 45, 200
　technology issues 43–4
　visualization/mindfulness 46
　working at depth 43
　working with stories 47
oracle cards 34
organizational Creative Counselling 201
outdoor settings *see* nature interventions
overanalysing/overthinking 18

pace and check 58–60, 71–2
Parenting Mental Health 26
Paylo, M. 204
Peacock, Caroline 109–10
peer support 197
percussion instruments 97
Perryman, K. 204, 205, 206
perspective (shifts in) 154–5
pet intervention 109–10
photographing work 159, 168–9
photos 34, 40
planned endings 162–3
poetry
　and embodiment/role play 101
　focusing on a theme 99
　mindful poetry 98–9
　three-line poem 98
　working with 100
Polyvagal Theory 59–60

Poquérusse, J. 203
positive thoughts garden 52–3
power animal 183
power five 184
prices 180–1
Priestley, Shelby 51–3
privacy during online counselling 44
puppets 123–7

rates 180–1
reflecting
　conversational writing 158
　influences on 149–52
　overview 147
　reflective writing 157
　role play 158
　through giving a title to
　　the creation 158
　through Mind, Body, Feelings and
　　Intuition (MBFI) 152–3
　using photography 159
relational depth in online counselling 43
religious symbols 33
repetition (use of) 101–2
resources
　carrying (mobile counsellor) 40
　different types of 33–5
　digital 40
　diversity in 35–6
　sourcing 32
　therapist's own 179
Rimmer, Gaynor 148, 173
role play
　in counselling room 100–2
　in online counselling 46
　reflecting using 158
Rosen, C. 206
Rouse, A. 206

Sagan, O. 203, 206
sand tray
　exploring using 142
　first session (case history) 19–20
　grounding work with sand
　　67–8, 141–2
　my journey in the sand
　　exercise 171–2
　types of 33, 40
　using for assessment 82

screaming 96
self-awareness 178–82
self-care 72–6, 188–92, 196
self-compassion 75, 107, 197
self-regulation 94–5
self-talk
   empowering 192–5
   negative 107
sensory overload 39
Shaheen-Zaffar, Yasmin 143–6
Sharpe, Evie 105–8
Sharpe, Lin 132–6
sketching 178
Slyter, M. 203
Smith, C. 206
sound
   favourite 184
   grounding using 94–5
   incorporating within other interventions 94–7
   memories of 92–3
   musical instruments 97
   and nervous system 94
   as part of client's creation 95–6
   power of 92
   screaming/wailing 96
   to send healing 96–7
   tuning in to 93–4
Spears, E. 203
Stepakoff, S. 203
Stevens, R. 203
stones 127–31
storage
   client's work 166, 180
   resources 37–9
strengths board 106–7
supervision 199–200
symbols/symbolism 33–4, 149, 151, 167–8

talking therapy (not always enough) 18
then and now exercise 171
therapeutic alliance 56
therapeutic journaling 110–14
therapy (being in and out of) 26
This Mum Runs 26
Thomas, V. 202
three-line poem 98

time boundaries 180
timeline tools 86–7, 169–70
titling the creation 158
Tools Timeline 86–7, 169–70
training 198–9
transient art 52
transport symbols 34
Treanor, A. 43
trigger evaluation 84
trust 203
Trzaska, J. 206
tuning in
   to creation 153–4
   to sound 93–4

unconscious (working directly with) 18
unplanned endings 163

validation of feelings 155–7
verbalizing emotions 18
virtual counselling *see* online counselling
visual journaling 112–14
visualizations
   creative visualization 132–7
   during online counselling 46
   grounding 64–5

wailing 96
waiting lists (statistics) 27
walk-and-talk counselling 47–9
walk-and-talk supervision 200
Watson, Rebecca 101–2
Westergaard, J. 202, 206
Whisenhunt, J. 203, 205, 206
Whose Voice Is That? exercise 107–8
wild play sessions 48–9
window of tolerance 204–5
Winston, C. 203
word cards 173
word focus 186
workplace (Creative Counselling in) 201
Worry Buddies 126–7

YesTribe 26